I loved this book! Let me tell you why. I am an overweight, forty-nine-year-old woman. I have been on every diet imaginable and have worked with a trainer, but I still did not lose weight. Needless to say, before today, I had been very discouraged and had given up. But today after reading this inspiring book, I am encouraged and highly motivated to exercise, eat correctly, and develop a healthy lifestyle for me!

—JAN DRAVECKY
WIFE OF FORMER MAJOR LEAGUE PITCHER DAVE DRAVECKY
AUTHOR, *A Joy I'd Never Known*

For years I've thought a personal trainer is a luxury reserved for only the rich and famous. *Fit Over 50* gives me all the benefits of a personal trainer for just the price of one book! Lorraine's advice and instructions are easy to understand, but just like with a pricey personal trainer's hands-on guidance, doing it takes commitment and *discipline.*

This book's message not only instructs, but it also motivates! Good health is more than diet and exercise; it also includes emotional, mental, physical, and spiritual aspects…and this book addresses all four. Lorraine doesn't pull any punches. She makes it clear that "no miracle cure exists."

I'm a management consultant, and I frequently advise my clients to encourage good health habits for their employees of all ages, because healthy employees are happier, have fewer absences, and are more productive. So there's a financial benefit in adopting the message of this book into your life, too.

I've known Lorraine since she was a teen, and one of the things I appreciate most about her is her high level of integrity. She is a living example of the message of this book. It's not just "feel good" advice but a message delivered with passion from a disciplined practitioner.

My advice is simple. Buy this book, read it, and live to experience and enjoy your dreams!

—GARY D. FOSTER
GARY D. FOSTER CONSULTING

I didn't know Lorraine could read my mind. *Of course* I hate exercise. *Of course* I hate vegetables and vitamin pills. By the way, I believe vitamin pills are DANGEROUS. My wife, Barb, has me take 20,765 pills every morning while she's in her rocking chair studying her Precept Bible Lesson for the Seattle Mariner wives she ministers to. Usually about pill number 20,763 I gag and cough. From the rocking chair I hear, "You should see how many pills I would like you to take!" Barb and I write marriage books, so I'm ever on the lookout for more material. What I want from Barb when I'm choking to death is "Ooohhh." *Period.* No commentary…no advice…no recrimination…just grace! Now is that too much to ask? I guess it is. Anyway I invented the "OH" principle, and I'll be sure to put it in my next book. I love the fact that Lorraine gives an old guy like me hope. She doesn't start me off with 887-pound barbells. She hands me a postcard and tells me to "be careful." Now *that* I can handle. You'll love her style, her honesty, and her amazing talent in getting old people like me to exercise.

—CHUCK SNYDER
COAUTHOR, *Incompatibility: Still Grounds for a Great Marriage*

Lorraine has written a book that is long overdue for those fifty and over. Having broken the fifty barrier myself, I was motivated after reading her book to make a better effort at getting fit. This book is a winner for my generation and will make anyone who reads it ready to hit the treadmill!

—STAN TOLER
AUTHOR AND PASTOR, OKLAHOMA CITY, OK

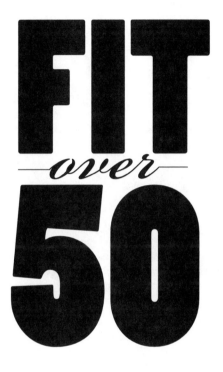

FIT
over
50

LORRAINE BOSSÉ-SMITH

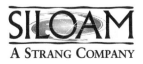

SILOAM
A STRANG COMPANY

Most STRANG COMMUNICATIONS/CHARISMA HOUSE/SILOAM/REALMS products are available at special quantity discounts for bulk purchase for sales promotions, premiums, fund-raising, and educational needs. For details, write Strang Communications/Charisma House/Siloam/Realms, 600 Rinehart Road, Lake Mary, Florida 32746, or telephone (407) 333-0600.

FIT OVER 50 by Lorraine Bossé-Smith
Published by Siloam
A Strang Company
600 Rinehart Road
Lake Mary, Florida 32746
www.siloam.com

Cover design by Justin Evans

Neither the publisher nor the author is engaged in rendering professional advice or services to the individual reader. The ideas, procedures, and suggestions in this book are not intended as a substitute for consulting with your physician. All matters regarding your health require medical supervision. Neither the author nor the publisher shall be liable or responsible for any loss or damage allegedly arising from any information or suggestion in this book.

While the author has made every effort to provide accurate telephone numbers and Internet addresses at the time of publication, neither the publisher nor the author assumes any responsibility for errors or for changes that occur after publication.

Library of Congress Cataloging-in-Publication Data
Bosse-Smith, Loraine, 1966-
  Fit over 50 / Lorraine Bosse-Smith.-- 1st ed.
      p. cm.
  Includes bibliographical references (p.   ).
  ISBN 1-59185-820-8 (paper back)
  1. Middle-aged persons--Health and hygiene. 2. Older people--Health and hygiene. 3. Physical fitnesss for middle-aged persons. 4. Physical fitness for older people. 5. Middle-aged persons--Nutrition. 6. Older people--Nutrition. I. Title: Fit over fifty. II. Title.
RA777.5.B68 2005
  613.7'044
                                    2005031352

First Edition

06 07 08 09 10 — 987654321
Printed in the United States of America

*I would like to dedicate this book
to the dearest couple I know…
Dallas and Opal Shafer.*

*You recently celebrated fifty years of marriage,
and more than three hundred people came to share in
your joy. We also came as a testimony of your faithful-
ness and love not only to each other but to Him.*

*Thank you for showing me the way and
for being a living example of the fact that
life really does just keep getting better with age!*

*With much love,
Lorraine*

Acknowledgments

I would like to thank every person who has allowed me to come into his or her life and make a contribution by teaching safe, effective ways to work out and stay healthy. I appreciate the trust you extend to me, and I am impressed with your dedication and commitment to taking care of the body you have been given. Especially to those over the age of fifty, you have truly touched my heart and blessed me richly. You inspire us all!

I would like to also extend gratitude to my church, Cornerstone Community Church, for their continued support and encouragement of my writing, speaking, and fitness endeavors. Cathy, in particular, you have lived out God's love in so many ways. You're awesome!

To my dear friends and family who helped me with editing, stories, support, and encouragement, thank you all for giving of yourselves and your time. I appreciate you and thank God for you! My list is too long to include everyone, but you know who you are, and I am truly blessed!

Jann Gentry once again provided her incredible photography talent to this book, and I can't thank her enough for not only being so professional and creative but also for having such a kind and loving spirit. Need a photographer? Check out www.janngentry.com.

To the models you find in this book, Marion and Tim, thank you for being real, living examples of the principles in this book and physically showing folks that they can do it, too! You are both beautiful people inside and out.

To the team at Siloam, I extend my appreciation for partnering with me on this important project. Thanks for all you do for His kingdom.

Contents

Table of Charts

Foreword

When I was in high school and college, I played football. I was always in good shape physically because I had coaches and trainers to help me. Their job was to make sure I ate right, trained hard, and stayed in tip-top condition. Being a good athlete is not a part-time job. Even though the sport I was playing took place only in the fall of each year, we still lifted weights, ran, wrestled, and worked out all year round to stay in good shape.

Although, at the time, I did not love that kind of discipline, it sure paid good dividends. I was never sick and always fit nicely into my clothes. To this very day I look back at those pictures and feel proud about the results I achieved in my personal life. I had no idea what was about to happen next.

As the years rolled along, my self-discipline got weaker and weaker. I had no one "standing over me" encouraging me to stay in good shape. I now realize how little I really knew about exercise and nutrition. When you have someone overseeing your workouts and your eating schedule, it becomes rather simple to keep up with them. You don't even have to think about it! I had to make a concentrated effort to get back into shape and to eat a good, healthy diet.

After turning fifty years old and being as active as I am, I began to realize the importance and necessity of staying healthy and mobile. I wanted someone to give me some guidance. So I turned to Lorraine Bossé-Smith. Lorraine gave me the needed insights to help me stay healthier. Her information is especially important for those of us in the baby-boomer generation as we get older. In my personal quest to remain healthy and fit, I found few books that actually focus on people our age who are still very active. I am grateful to Lorraine and her insights on practical ways to stay fit and yet keep up with a busy lifestyle.

As you read this book you are going to find simple ways to bring back the youth and vitality you either once knew or long to have. The human body is a great machine. All it needs is a little attention. I am grateful I found the information I needed in this book!

—ROBERT A. ROHM, PHD
PRESIDENT, PERSONALITY INSIGHTS, INC.
ATLANTA, GA

Introduction

Life's Best Chapter

I have a dear friend in Gallatin, Tennessee (near Nashville), who is retired. Rather than calling this time in his life his "golden years," as so many in the media refer to it, he has opted to call it "life's best chapter." In fact, he was so passionate about this life-changing event that he wrote a book by the same name some years ago (New Hope Publishers).

Having the door closed on his corporate career and spending more time at home wasn't just an adjustment for *him*—his wife found the transition difficult as well. He was on her turf now! His book shares some very funny and sweet stories about the transition. He found that he needed to identify with something other than work, and she learned that she needed to change her routine to accommodate him. Easier said than done.

Perhaps you have been there and done that. I know I completely related to that story, even though I'm not retired. I left corporate America to start my own business in 1997. I soon found myself going through similar feelings of isolation. My home was now my office, so I had to learn to create boundaries and adjust to all the changes of being a one-woman show. Then in 1998 things got even more complicated when I married and began working with my husband out of the home.

My friend's book was a great help, and you might enjoy it, too. It was just re-released under the title *How to Retire Without Retreating* by Johnnie Godwin, published by Barbour Publishing.[1]

Life Changes

As you begin to approach the fifty-plus mark (or begin to pass it), it is not just your career that changes but your *entire* life. Being fifty-plus certainly is not what it was years ago. In fact, many people today switch careers at this critical junction and begin doing something they enjoy rather than "having to do it for the money." Nonetheless, the body changes, the mind alters, and the energy diminishes. The facts are that 30 percent of the aging process will happen no matter what you do.[2]

We have control over 70 percent of the aging process.

It begins when we're in our twenties, believe it or not. I remember being at the doctor's office for my annual checkup at the age of twenty-six. I was reading a pamphlet that notified me I was beginning the "dying process." Excuse me? It turns out that up until our twenties, we are creating new skin, new cells, growth, and so on. But after that point, our body starts to prepare for death. This was not what I wanted to hear at twenty-six! In fact, I am not sure I ever really want to hear that.

The good news is that we do have control over about 70 percent of the process.[3] Whew! How we will age and what our "next chapter" will look like has much to do with how we live life today. Do you want it to be the best chapter ever? If so, then your health will be paramount.

You inspire me!

Right about now, you're probably saying, "You're only in your thirties—what do you know about getting old?" Well, it's true that I am only in my early forties and have not yet come to the stage in life you are living. However, I have researched, studied, trained, and taken a genuine interest in the fifty-plus age group.

I am inspired and encouraged by you. When we were younger, things came a little easier. But when the body ages, the same things take a little more effort. I am so very impressed with the hard work people such as you give to life. By watching you and learning about you, I completely understand the importance of doing it right today to ensure a healthier tomorrow. By taking training courses and educating myself, I can help folks in the next stages of life make it better.

My passion and desire is to improve the quality of your life. I have coached, trained, and taught many folks over the age of fifty, and I hope you will permit me to join your journey to better health.

It's all about choices

So what is all the hubbub about health and fitness anyway? You can't watch television, read a newspaper or magazine, or simply drive down the road without seeing and hearing something about health. In years past, it really wasn't discussed much. During my parents' generation, they actually thought smoking was good for you! We have certainly come a long way and have obtained incredible amounts of helpful information regarding health.

The challenge now is how to best approach it. Many fads are out there with extraordinary claims: lose weight fast without exercising, be healthy and eat whatever you want, and the like. These claims are all marketing and sales hype. Please don't fall for the "sounds too good to be true" fad, because it probably is not true!

Ever hear of Skinny Cow products? They are ice cream bars and sandwiches that are "good for you." Many of my clients have switched to these instead of regular ice cream. Occasionally, I guess this is OK, but have you ever read what's actually in a Skinny Cow product? One of their latest fat-free, carb-free products is nothing but chemicals! I don't know what they are made of. I can't pronounce most of the ingredients.

Here's a quick nugget: *when they take one thing out, they replace it with something else.* For instance, if it's fat free, then they will increase the sugar for taste. If it is low carb, then most likely they have added more fat. In this case they have replaced nutrients with chemicals that are not good for the body at all.

If it sounds too good to be true, it probably is.

The real truth is that good health is a day-by-day commitment of eating right and exercising. Period. No miracle cure exists. The good news is that it's simple to do: burn more calories than you take in. Unfortunately, even though most people have heard this advice, many are not living by this principle.

Alarming statistics

Our country is suffering from obesity at a startling rate. A recent study by the *Archives of Internal Medicine* cited data showing that about two-thirds of U.S. adults—131 million people—are overweight.[4] The Aerobics and Fitness Association of America has found that 80 percent of Americans are not getting enough exercise on a weekly basis to have any health benefit.[5] One million people die of a heart attack each year. For the first time in our history, women are dying at the same rate as men.[6]

All of this means that our country is very unhealthy, and an unhealthy life is costly to us all.

What is poor health costing *you?* Poor health can result in:

- Low energy
- Restless nights/lack of sleep
- Depression/anxiety
- Decreased productivity
- Aches and pains
- Unhappiness/mood swings
- Frequent sickness/illness
- Excessive hair loss
- Weight gain
- Diseases such as coronary heart disease, cancer, diabetes, emphysema, and osteoporosis

- Sexual dysfunction
- Premature death

Being overweight in particular causes you to be subject to a number of ailments that you'd likely never get if you were slimmer. Did you know that 70 percent of all illnesses and injuries in America are preventable?[7] The best way to avoid the doctor's office is to exercise and eat right—and this applies to any age group.

Seasoned veterans

As we get older, we simply need to modify what we do and how we do it.

I love teaching my fitness classes here in Southern California to a group of people over the age of fifty. I hesitate to call them "seniors" because they're far from the image that I get with the word *senior:* someone sitting in a rocking chair watching life pass them by. They certainly have seniority over me with life experience and wisdom, which is one of the reasons I love interacting with them so much. And they have a wealth of knowledge to share.

My class members work extremely hard. They are so committed to exercising because they know they need to. It is not a "want to" anymore but a "must do." They have learned through time the benefits of a healthy lifestyle. They truly want to avoid an unhealthy life today so that they can have a better tomorrow.

In *Fit Over 50* I will be calling this group "seasoned veterans."

BENEFITS OF A HEALTHY LIFESTYLE

Every seasoned veteran will receive many benefits from living a healthy lifestyle:

- Being active will improve the quality of your sleep.

- Weight-bearing exercise will increase your bone density and reduce your chances of osteoporosis.

- Working your heart will decrease your blood pressure and improve your circulation.

- Including cardiovascular exercise at least three times a week at a moderate intensity level will lower your cholesterol levels.

- Participating in active programs will keep you mentally alert and sharpen your senses.

- Exercising and eating right will minimize aches and pains.

- Stretching will improve joint movement and improve overall mobility, preventing unnecessary injuries.

- Staying fit will give you more energy and help you be more productive (yes, at home counts).

- Exercising will reduce stress and depression.

- Living an active lifestyle will help keep you at a healthy weight, which in turn can eliminate back pain.

- Being in shape will help you feel better about yourself and give you a more positive outlook on life.

- Finally, the healthier you are, the less likely you are to get sick or incur illness.[8]

This list should excite you! These are very tangible, real benefits that are available to you with a little effort, commitment, and time.

The folks who attend my classes for the reasons above really inspire me. It gives me hope to know that if I do the right things today I can end up in as good of shape and health as they are in their best chapter of life.

Every once in a while, a young whippersnapper (thirties or forties) gal will join our seasoned veterans' class. Although she may be expecting rocking chairs and walkers, what she ends up getting is a phe-nomenal cardiovascular and muscle-sculpting workout that is really fun. Nothing gives me greater joy than to see my seventy-year-olds outperforming a younger person—all with a big smile! They can do this because they have been working on improving their health.

The best way to avoid the doctor's office is to exercise and eat right.

And better health is within your reach, too. It is never too late to embark on a healthier path.

It's never too late

Our bodies are amazing. We can abuse them by doing all the wrong things, but once we stop, they heal.

My mother had smoked cigarettes since she was a teenager. Remember, back then, they were told cigarettes were actually good for you. After my dad died of cancer, my mother began questioning her habits. Her first few attempts to quit were brutal. She was grumpy, angry, and a bear to live with. I know, I was there! She had been trying to quit for the wrong reasons: other people. When she finally decided that she wanted to be healthy, she was actually able to quit. In a year's time her lungs were almost clear. Her body was healing. Later in life she took it a step further to eat better and exercise, and her body responded by being in the best shape she had ever been—and she was in her sixties!

So don't think you are too old or too set in your ways to make a change. Small steps can get you there. You can do it. You must do it. And your body (and God) will be there for you.

Grow better, not old

You've probably heard people quote Robert Browning, who began one of his poems by saying, "Grow old along with me, the best is yet to be." How romantic and sentimental. Yet in order to make this a reality, you must make your health a priority.

My dear friends Dallas and Opal celebrated their fiftieth anniversary in 2004. Personally, I think they deserve a medal on top of the party they had! But when I told them my thoughts, they disagreed. Their comment was that it couldn't be fifty years already. They were just having too much fun.

I believe their secret is continually being active. They have not allowed age to be an excuse. They still get out and ride their bikes, hike, and travel. Their intensity level has certainly changed, but their passion and zest for a full life has not. Their motivation for all of this is to grow old together. They married for life, and they want that life together to last as long as possible. And they want it to be enjoyable.

Even if you're not married, you have friends and family who want you to be around a very long time. Besides doing it for your own good, getting healthy is a great gift to give others.

The gift of good health

Fit Over 50 is my gift to you as you enter a new chapter of life. I know you desire a full life as well. This book is designed to educate you on what a healthy life is without all the hubbub. It will help you create meal plans that are balanced and nutritious, not to mention realistic. It will not let you off the hook for exercising, but it will give you strategies for working out that are appropriate for your stage of life (forty-five to fifty-five, fifty-six to sixty-five, and sixty-six and older).

Through these pages I will be your personal trainer, here to help you reach your goal of better health because I want you to be around for a long time, too!

YOUR PERSONAL TRAINER

Speaking of personal training, let me quickly share a little about myself in order for you to know with whom you are working. And by the way, I am very honored that you have selected me.

I've been an active person my entire life. I took very good care of my physical condition, but major stresses of life back in 1997 forced me to redefine my health habits even further. I was not caring for my entire self. (Read my first book, *A Healthier, Happier You: 101 Steps for Lessening Stress* for more on that story.) Out of necessity and for my own well-being, I began digging deeper into the health and fitness industry.

I was so impressed with what I learned and how it brought me to total health that I became a certified personal trainer. My goal and desire since then has been to help others improve the quality of their lives, just as mine had been improved through proper nutrition and exercise.

I have been teaching an array of fitness classes for years now. I even opened my own private studio to train clients toward better health. I speak to groups and teach wellness workshops across the country. I started writing books in hopes of reaching even more people; perhaps you have read my previous book *Finally FIT! Customizing Fitness to Your Personality Type.* In that book, you discover how your unique personality influences your workout.

How about some personal details so you can get to know me just a little more? I love music, playing tennis, hiking, watching movies, and being with friends. I live with my husband and our two cats in beautiful southern California.

As a reader of *Fit Over 50* you have just entered into a coaching/personal training relationship with me. Thank you for your trust and desire to improve. I am excited to be working together with you, and I think you will be pleased with your results.

Be determined and deliberate

In order to move toward better health, though, you must not only make a commitment; you must also take action. This is where a lot of people can get stuck.

Marion is a great example. She turned sixty in 2005. She had always been a jogger, but years ago she was told she would not be able to run again because of her fibromyalgia. The prognosis was that she would basically suffer and be in pain for the rest of her life. This discouraged her, and she really missed running. But instead of letting it overwhelm her, she decided to take charge of her life. Despite what doctors had said, she made getting healthy a goal so that she could possibly run again.

When she came to me, she had already drastically changed her diet. She was avoiding foods that made her feel bad, and she was making healthy choices. With my coaching and guidance, she recently began running again. She started off slow and has been able to go farther and faster than she imagined.

Instead of focusing on what she could not do, she started taking steps that she could take. Rather than simply talk about it, she did it. Marion is in better shape now than she was in her forties. She is strong, lean, and healthy—not to mention pain-free!

Please do not settle for poor health and accept it as "good enough." I am so very pleased that you have made the first step by purchasing this book. Your next step is to read it and begin to apply it.

Keep these things in mind as you do:

1. Remember that you want to learn how to live a healthier life. Do not get so caught up in how the message is delivered, but rather concentrate on what it can do for you.

2. Keep your mind open to new information, concepts, and strategies. Even if you have heard or read some of the details in this book before, apply them in a different manner.

3. Give everything some time to sink in before you say yea or nay and make your final decision on how it will work for you.

4. Take the information provided and build upon it, making it personal and suitable for your particular situation. Make it work for you.

5. You will find what you seek. If you think fitness and health is a bunch of hogwash, then you will not discover all the gems found within this book's pages. If,

on the other hand, you look for positive ways to
improve the quality of your life, then you will find
outstanding ways to change your life. You decide what
you get out of this book and if you will succeed.

As your personal trainer, I look forward to providing you with
information that will help you make better decisions regarding your
health. You've made a commitment, are willing to take action, and are
proceeding with an open mind—so let's get started! Get ready for a
healthier you. I pray I am truly able to improve the quality of your life
and that you enjoy our journey together. Thank you for selecting me
to be a part of your life. I am honored. Remember, with God all things
are possible!

FIT

Section One

It's Up to You!

50

Chapter One

Time to Get Fit!

Recently I had a flat tire in Los Angeles. My perfectly smooth ride suddenly became unbalanced and dangerous. Plus, the Los Angeles freeway is not safe even at the best of times! I was in the far left lane trying to move over to the right lane, praying all the while that I would make it. I felt desperate. By the time I managed to get the car off the freeway, I was emotionally and mentally exhausted. I didn't like the feeling of my car being out of balance like that, and I couldn't wait to get an inflated tire back on my car.

You may have experienced a similar situation at some point—hopefully not in the heart of Los Angeles! What a bumpy, uncomfortable, and unstable ride it is when just one tire is either out of balance or flat.

Know when to say yes and when to say no.

Our bodies are no different. God made us with four aspects of our being: emotional, mental, physical, and spiritual. They are all vital to our overall health. If we truly want to be healthy, then we need to work on all four to ensure we have complete balance or a "smooth ride." Riding around with three good tires is not good enough. Unfortunately, many people sacrifice their health to the point where one tire is completely gone. You cannot expect your ride to be smooth if you are ignoring a flat tire.

Just like your car, your body cannot perform properly without all four tires fully inflated. Balance is the key.

When you ignore one of your aspects, or "tires," you are a blowout waiting to happen! If you ignore your unbalanced health by not doing anything about it, it will catch up with you.

The amazing thing about concentrating on one's health is that when you correct your physical health, the other three areas (emotional, mental, and spiritual health) automatically improve. The healthier your body becomes, the healthier the rest of you becomes—and I want you to be healthy!

Balance is the key.

Just because you are retired or nearing retirement doesn't mean you walk away from principles you learned in your youth. Some retirees take not having to work to an extreme and stop working on everything, including their health. I believe it is even more critical at the fifty-plus mark to monitor one's health and work on improving it.

Take a look around you, and you will see many retired folks spending their "free" days at the doctor's office or in line at the pharmacy. Is that how you want to spend your time? I wish more than that for you. I would like to see you enjoy a healthy lifestyle that allows you to do the things you have always dreamed of.

My father never had that chance. He died of cancer at the very young age of fifty-two. I remember him speaking of the day when he would get to travel and see the United States, but his day never came. His premature death is a very good reminder that we do not know how much time we have here on earth. I believe that we should make the most of it, give our all, and love all. Although none of us have guarantees, living a healthy lifestyle is certainly going to help us enjoy the time we do have on earth.

A healthy lifestyle is not something we're born with. Rather, it is something we must create. And once again, it involves some balancing on our part. In order to improve our physical body or health, we must address our nutrition, our cardiovascular health (heart health), our muscles (for bone health), and our flexibility. Isn't it interesting that these are like four more tires? All four must be maintained properly to create good health. Even though some people are born with tendencies toward eating healthier foods and others inherit a fondness for exercise, all of us make daily choices that impact our health.

I know about a man who was an entrepreneur who enjoyed success at every level. Everything he touched seemed to go perfectly. He was in control of his life and liked it that way. But one day, some years ago now, he received a surprise: he suffered a mild stroke. Having never experienced failure before and feeling totally out of control, he gave up living on that very day. Although doctors strongly encouraged him to take care of himself, because doing so would improve his condition, he chose not to do anything positive. He ate the wrong things and did not care for his body. He died recently, in his eighties, in pain and quite miserable. He lived with the consequences of bad decisions.

Don't make the same mistake. Weigh your options and consider the costs carefully.

OPPORTUNITY SCALE

You have made a decision to read this book. I appreciate it and hope each page makes a difference in your life. But as you read this, you are unable to do anything else. (OK, unless you are a super-duper multitasker who can do twelve things at once.) For this moment at least you have chosen not to wash the car, walk the dog, call a friend, grocery shop, iron clothes, work on the car, play golf or tennis, or whatever. You said no to everything else when you said yes to reading.

Without knowing it, each of us weighs out our options every moment of every day. We evaluate the costs associated with them, as well. If you opted to miss your granddaughter's first birthday because you wanted to read my book instead, I would say you did not think through the cost. A first birthday is something that can never occur again. On the other hand, my book will be here waiting for you. I would not expect anyone to pay that price, but amazingly, people often do choose the wrong thing.

Chart 1.1—Opportunity Scale

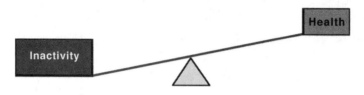

In order to become healthy, you must be willing to make some tough decisions. You will need to weigh the costs. Sometimes they seem insignificant, but they can add up to be very expensive. The man in the above story did not want to pay the price of changing his lifestyle. He refused to change. As a consequence, he had horrible health. He had to rely on others to care for him. An immediate cost may sting a little, but the long-term value of good health cannot be matched. You must commit to making better choices.

Commitment

Past generations seemed to have the philosophy that once a person retired, he or she retired from everything: work *and* working out. Today, people are more health conscious because they are living longer and want a better quality of life.

Enough information is out there to support the theory that if you eat right and exercise you will live a better life. In fact, in January 2005 the federal government released new standards for us. To summarize their lengthy findings: eat less and exercise more. Wow. I hope you were sitting down while you read that! It's not earth-shattering, is it? Therefore, even those who retire are now committing to exercise. What an exciting day we live in!

My friend Johnnie, whom I mentioned in the introduction, is totally committed to his health. He has been jumping rope every day, without fail, since he was young. After that, he does some sit-ups and push-ups. He has been doing this longer than I have been alive. And do you know what? He is in great shape! Even though he is nearing seventy, he has the energy of a thirty-year-old. He hasn't done anything extraordinary, but he *has* done it faithfully, day by day. Consistency is paramount, but it is not the only thing.

If you eat right and exercise you will live a better life.

The body is an amazing thing. Remember the story of my mother's smoking addiction? She created massive damage to her lungs for over thirty years, but after she quit smoking, her body restored and repaired her lungs within a year. Some scar tissue may have remained, but she was healthy again. If you have made some poor health choices in the past, they are in the past. Today is a new day! Today is the day when you can make steps toward better health, and I am here to help.

WHAT TO EXPECT IN THIS BOOK

In chapter two, you will have the opportunity to give some thought to your life and what you want out of it. I am talking about setting some goals. *I gave that up when I retired*, you might be thinking. Well, you know better. You know that much wasn't accomplished at work without goals. Someone set the target in front of you, and you aimed for it. Our health is no different. If we do not know what we are shooting for, we will not hit it.

Chapter three will address the aging process. My goal is to be realistic as well as sensitive to the other aspects of the aging process outside of the physical changes that occur. We will look at the emotional adjustments you have been making and will continue to make. Dallas and Opal often mention how sharp their minds are—as if they were twenty. But the body just doesn't cooperate. This can cause very real frustrations and possibly lead to depression if not handled properly. We must include this in the total picture for you to truly gain whole health.

Chapter four will give you some incredible insight into your heart health and how you can monitor your own exercise based on your physical condition, age, and objectives. I don't like the standard formulas that are typically used for such things. Instead, I will tell you how to monitor your own breathing. It is *you* we are concerned about, not some test subject. The goal: to make your time spent exercising count! If you put the time in, you should get the health benefits.

Knowledge is power.

Remember, the body was designed to move, but the heart needs to be challenged in order to remain strong. If you don't know how your body works, any time you spend in exercise may be wasted. Certainly, getting out and moving is good for you, but if you truly want to improve your cardiovascular capacity and reduce your chances of heart disease, then you must work the body hard enough. Knowledge is power!

Then in chapter five you will learn about weight-bearing exercise and how critical this is to your overall health. As you get older, you want to be able to function in life with little pain and without injury. I will help you outline a plan that sets you up for success. You will devise a routine that challenges you but does not hurt you. I think we all need to be pushed, but we still need to be safe. If it is not safe, people get injured and then they can't work out. This creates frustration and discouragement. I want to foster a positive environment for you.

Chapters six, seven, and eight are specifically written for the three stages of life I am addressing in this book. They are where the "rubber meets the road," and they will provide you with exercise suggestions for your age group. You will be given an exercise guide and stretches to perform. Since a picture speaks a thousand words, you will have photos to help you along. Marion and Tim were gracious enough to help model proper technique for you. They are both in their sixties, and if they can do it, so can you!

The last two chapters help you discover what a well-balanced diet is and how to create an appropriate meal plan that fits you. Check out the Daily Healthy Life Journal in chapter ten. It will help you work on balance every day.

BEFORE YOU GET STARTED

Something else that will really help you is a visit to your doctor's office before embarking on any new exercise program. Get a complete physical, and ask how any prescription drugs you are currently taking will alter your heart rate and how you should adapt. Even if you have exercised at some point in the past, it might be a good idea to get an overall checkup before starting a new exercise program.

Your doctor will evaluate your health condition, check your cholesterol levels, and take your blood pressure. All of this is important data to know. Knowing your blood pressure and cholesterol levels is more than just good information to have; it will give you a benchmark to measure your progress. After six months of sticking to your new workout, get them rechecked. I can almost bet you will see positive, encouraging results!

One of my cycling class members came to me because he was discouraged by his high cholesterol levels. His doctor told him that he had better do something or else. He is happily married and wanted to continue living that life, so he tried cycling. I told him that if he joined me three days a week and worked out at the proper intensity levels while cycling that he would see a change in three months. He did. In fact, his cholesterol levels were so low that his doctor wondered what drug he was taking. The body is an amazing thing, but it needs your help.

It's time to get fit!

Of course, all my advice and counsel will not change a thing if you are not willing to apply it. The most important factor of your entire exercise program is you. Whatever your age today, there is no time like the present to get started. The time is now to get fit, healthy, robust, well, in shape, able-bodied—whatever you want to call it. Are you ready and willing? Let's get started!

Chapter Two

You Make the Difference

I have been writing since I was a child. In a scrapbook somewhere (which I started before it was a hip trend) I have the very first poem I ever wrote, misspellings and all. As an adult I have created my own workbooks and training programs, and I have written countless articles for magazines and newspapers across the country.

Writing a book, however, is an entirely different process. Publishers have very specific goals for you. They determine how many words you must type and by when. Talk about a bull's-eye target to hit! However, without it, I might deliver something too short or too verbose. And I might not provide it in time for them to print it. Having the target in front of me kept me focused, on task, and accountable.

Our lives are no different. We have things we want to do but somehow we get off track—if we don't have a plan or target in front of us. We were designed to focus forward, toward something. We get in trouble when we drift aimlessly and do whatever feels good for the moment.

Life has enough obstacles to throw your way—you have lived through many, I'm sure—so plan where you want to go and how you will get there. Develop strategies to overcome the challenges when they come. Be ready!

What Is *Your* Goal?

Throughout your life you have most likely learned the importance of planning. The old saying is still relevant: "No one plans to fail but always will if they fail to plan."

Every aspect of our lives—including fitness and health—requires planning. You must have a map if you hope to arrive at your destination. It's no different when your destination or goal is good health. You must know your exact location *today* in order to arrive at *tomorrow* with the health you hope to obtain. Goal setting is the key.

I'm not talking about desires, although most of us have them. Desires are things we talk about wanting but never really do anything about. I personally *desire* to be a rock star. I think we all have a star inside of us dying to come out. I would love to bounce and jump around on stage, banging out a great, high-energy tune, making people smile. But I do not sing (other than at church on Sunday), nor do I take lessons. Therefore it is not a *goal* because I have not taken any action toward it. Goals require action. *Dreams* are not goals, either. We tend to feel more passionate about our dreams than we do about our desires, but a dream does not become a goal until we take steps toward it.

No one plans to fail.

I believe that today, more than any other time in history, health is a goal for most people. Thanks to medical science we have a longer life expectancy and improved living conditions. However, most people don't change their habits or behaviors when it comes to a healthy lifestyle. "Why can't I eat fast food all the time?" "Do I really have to exercise?" American culture has taught us for years that we can have it "our way." But when it comes to our health, we need to do it *God's* way, which involves discipline and work.

We can't expect different results if we keep doing the same thing we have always done. Instead of creating frustration and hopelessness, decide to take action toward your goal of good health and commit to it. This will actually help you achieve it, no matter what your age.

Remember Dallas and Opal? Their motivation for doing the right things is to live a very long, healthy, and happy life together. The first fifty years have gone by so quickly, and they are looking forward to the future with hope!

What is your goal? What has motivated you to pick up this book? Whatever it is, you must be willing to do whatever it takes to accomplish your goal.

BE SMART WITH YOUR GOALS

Goals define what we want to achieve. They direct our energy, determine our priorities, and keep us motivated and on the right track. All goals are not created equal, however. It is one thing to *set* goals; it is a completely different thing to *achieve* them. I want to help you obtain what you want: good health.

Let's talk about your health goal for a minute. If you haven't given it much thought yet, this chapter will guide you through an excellent process of determining what you really want and how to obtain it. You don't have to share this with anyone, but I do encourage you to disclose it to a person close to you. When we actually speak our goals verbally to another person we tend to make a deeper commitment to them. And a loved one or close friend can be a great support system and accountability partner.

Your health goal needs to conform to the following list of criteria. As you develop your goal, be sure it incorporates each of these areas. If it doesn't, you will need to rework your goal in order to ensure you will reach your target. Your goal must be SMART:

Chart 2.1—SMART Goals

• **S**pecific	Gives us a target/direction to focus our energy and activity
• **M**easurable	Measures progress and knows when we achieve the goal
• **A**ctionable	Requires some kind of action (required to achieve anything)
• **R**ealistic	Provides motivation through faith that we can/will achieve our goal
• **T**imed	Time specific; accountability; keeps us on track

My fitness classes tease that the word *focus* will be on my headstone. I use the word often in classes to help people stay on track with the particular goal we may have at that time. SMART goal setting brings into focus where you want to go, providing a clear target to hit.

Take your health goal, and get real with it. Write it down. Then spend time looking at each of these elements and make sure you have addressed each one with your written goal. Remember to be specific with what you are trying to accomplish. The more details you can include, the more you will know what you are attempting to do and what will be required of you. Besides, with clarity comes focus.

Let me give you an example. A client of mine came to me after being on the Atkins diet for six months. He lost a ton of weight quickly, but he felt horrible and had no energy. He lost so much muscle that he couldn't even push his lawn mower. (NOTE: Please be careful with extreme diets of this nature. Many programs eliminate carbohydrates from your diet, and carbs are a crucial and essential element to your health. Carbs are your body's main source of energy. See chapter nine for more on this.) This client was only in his sixties and was very concerned about what had happened. To start him on the road to recovery, we sat down and set some goals according to the SMART model.

First, we made a *specific* outline of what he wanted to do. He didn't want to compete in a muscleman contest, but he did want to care for his home and family. He still enjoyed being active in the community and working his business. We decided we would concentrate on muscle strengthening.

In order to make it *measurable*, we found out what weight he was able to lift and recorded it. We would then be able to see progress. He would work with me for a set period of time and then continue lifting on his own at home—this was the *actionable* part (the A in SMART). When time came to reevaluate him, we found that he had gained not only muscle strength but also core strength. He had more energy and did not feel run down. It worked! All he had to do was continue to maintain.

When we set the reevaluation time, we made sure that we were being *realistic* with his schedule. Make sure your goals are realistic, too, so you will set yourself up for success. Set goals that challenge you, certainly, but make sure they are actually attainable as well. We all do better when we can celebrate a victory, even if it is a small one.

My client's goal worked not only because it was specific, measurable, actionable, and realistic, but also because it was *timed*. Your goal needs to have a deadline. It has been said that a goal without a deadline is just a dream. If we put everything off until tomorrow, our goals will never become reality. A deadline creates a sense of pressure and helps us gain the momentum we need to take steps toward the final goal. Give yourself a realistic time frame to achieve your goal, but give yourself a deadline.

Be honest with your fitness goals as you write them out. Perhaps you want to lose ten pounds or gain muscle mass. Maybe you want to just tone up and stay about the same weight but hope to drop a dress size or two. You decide, and be sure to write them out. Those who write out their goals are ten times more successful at achieving them than those who do not.[1] This is the first step in making your dreams of a healthy life a reality.

Go over, go around, or go through

A fitness magazine once interviewed me to tell my story. I had to pause a moment to determine what would sum up my life. One word came to mind: *obstacles*. One recurrent theme in my life has been encountering challenges, some that I have created and others that have been thrown at me by others. Nonetheless, I had to decide at an early age that I would not let them stop me. With God's help, I would overcome the obstacles in my path.

So it is with you. To think you will never encounter any difficulties with your new health goal is sticking your head in the sand. In order to keep going toward your healthy future, be proactive. Do your best to anticipate the obstacles you may encounter along the way and the resistance you will face. Create a plan for how you will go over, around, or through those obstacles, but don't let them defeat you!

What if one of the obstacles is yourself? You are not alone. Everyone at one time or another is his or her own worst enemy with either negative self-talk or excuse making (otherwise called procrastination). That's why this chapter is so very important for you. The key to overcoming procrastination is to create a strong "why," a strong purpose. Knowing the reason you need to reach your goal will give you leverage to break bad habits and move past procrastination. Step by step you will get there!

When I start working with my training clients, I have them write down what they believe their biggest obstacle will be to achieving their fitness goal. The funniest one I have read yet is Mexican food! Most people list time and money (or lack thereof) as their greatest challenges. I will address time in a minute, but I want to be sensitive to your financial status. I have met many seasoned veterans who are living on a fixed income. Their options are more limited due to their income, but I want to encourage you that good health does not have to be expensive. Read on, and you will discover ways to improve your health right at home.

Your current health may even be an obstacle for you. It may be limiting what you can and can't do. Joint pain, muscle fatigue, mental fogginess, and lower energy are all real and will require some adjustment on your part. However, chapters six, seven, and eight of this book will give you ideas by age group. If you are younger but require special treatment due to your existing health condition, I encourage you to view chapters seven and eight for unique ways to exercise without hurting yourself. The goal is to improve your health, not make it worse.

Take a minute to jot down anything you think may get in your way. Don't get hung up on the list, but know it exists. Think of it as seeing the hazards in the road. By identifying the roadblocks, you can create a course that avoids them or minimizes their negative impact.

RTP

OK, now onto a time management tool called RTP. The letters stand for *resources, time,* and *people.* If you are like many other people, you may have listed *time* as one of your greatest obstacles. Even though you may actually have more time than in years past, isn't it amazing how all those hours get filled up? Whatever stage of life you happen to be in, time management is a key to exercise.

Everything we do requires resources, time, and people, and when we outline our needs in these three areas in advance we are more equipped to successfully reach our goals. You may already do this in your mind when managing your time on a day-to-day basis, but it's important to apply it to your health goal right now. Let's take the example of a cruise to Mexico. The RTP for this trip would look something like this:

Resources

- Tickets
- Passport
- Money
- Clothes
- Hat, sunglasses, and sunscreen
- Transportation to and from ship
- CD or DVD to learn Spanish

Time

- Three months to plan the trip
- Three months of practicing Spanish
- Block of time for the cruise (three days, five days, seven days, etc.)
- Driving time to and from cruise ship or port of call

People

- Travel agency
- Cruise line
- Travel companion
- Friends or family to watch your home, check your mail, and feed pets

Did I forget anything?

I have shown you how the RTP system helps you think through

everything you need to reach a goal. It can help you reach your health goal, too. Draw out your own health RTP right now. A simple piece of paper with three columns will do. Will you need to purchase hand weights or an actual weight-lifting machine? Will you need new shoes? Will you need to join a gym, or will you purchase your own cardio equipment? Will you hire a personal trainer?

This exercise is another great way to determine what you can do to either prevent the obstacles or overcome them. It will take only a minute, but it can make a huge difference.

Break it down

Understanding the resources, time, and people it will take to achieve your goal is one thing. Actually making it fit into your schedule is quite another! Most of us are not able to take something off our plate just because we add something new.

Take writing this book, for instance. I wish I could tell you I got to take a year off from everything else to write. But that could not be further from the truth. In order to have this book published, I had to find time to write within my existing schedule. I was given a firm deadline from my publisher, but to reach that final goal I found it helpful to break down how much I would do on a monthly, weekly, and daily basis. We can apply the process I used in writing this book to the health goal you have in mind.

The publisher gave me a total word count goal for the book. For you, the goal might be the number of pounds you want to lose. I then divided this word count number, which felt overwhelming at times, by the number of days I had to write. You would divide your total weight loss goal by the number of pounds that are healthy to lose each week (1 to 3, depending upon your gender). I counted on only four days a week to write, instead of five, to allow for "crazy" days. You might give yourself extra time to take into account any regular appointments or upcoming trips.

I arrived at a word count goal that I needed to reach each day to stay on schedule to meet my deadline. I then blocked out the appropriate amount of time each day to write those words, based on my typing speed. You can block out your workout days.

If you are like many of the retired seasoned veterans I work with, you have a packed schedule of babysitting grandchildren, serving on boards, volunteering in the community, *and* all the necessities of life (grocery shopping, house cleaning, car maintenance, and the like). In the midst of your full calendar, please carve out time for your health.

Know Your Energy Cycle

An excellent tool to chart out your peak energy times of the day in order to capitalize on them is what I call an energy graph. By using this graph, I have learned that my best creative time is in the afternoons, so I try to do all my other work in the mornings. Take a moment to draw out your energy cycle on the graph provided. If you have charted it before, chart how you feel now and compare it. It might be interesting to see how you have changed. To determine the best time to work out, notice the time of day when you have the most energy and the time when you are most tired.

Peak productivity times are when we are at our most energetic. By understanding when we are at our most productive levels, we can schedule certain events—such as workouts—at those times. Respect, protect, and direct your energy levels and peak productivity times.

Most of the seasoned veteran classes I teach are late morning. That might be a good time for you, too. You can get going in the morning and then go through the rest of the day feeling great. What works best for you?

Using the chart below, make an X to record your energy level at different times throughout the day. Then draw a line from X to X to map your energy level throughout the day. NOTE: Monitor a few days to get an accurate picture before you schedule your workout time. Chart your peak times and low times.

Chart 2.2-Energy Graph

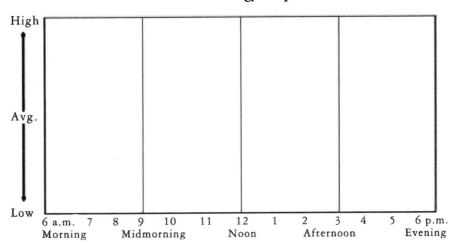

Even if you already know whether you are a morning person or an evening person, it can be quite insightful to see your energy levels throughout the day. If you use this information to customize your day to your energy flow, you will find that you are much more productive. In regards to your health, it will certainly ensure that you have the energy to work out.

Committing without getting committed!

Your energy will get you only so far. And every day is different. Some days you may actually have more energy while other days you just don't have it. Those are the days when commitment will pull you through.

Your goal to uphold and improve your health is something you do for yourself and for those you love. If you give and give but do not tend to your own needs, especially physical ones, you will actually end up hurting the ones you love by having poor health. If your true motivation is to give to others, then start by taking care of yourself. Commit to your health instead of getting committed! It's a much better option.

The best way to do this is to first love yourself. Remember, God loved you so much that He gave His one and only Son. If God loves you this much, you are worth something. You are valuable. Take care of yourself.

SET BOUNDARIES

Another way of keeping yourself in balance is to set boundaries. This requires learning to say one simple word: *no*. For such a small word, *no* can be extremely difficult for some people to say. However, learning to set boundaries will improve your emotional and mental health, not to mention freeing up time for your physical health. A great book on this subject is *Boundaries* by Drs. Cloud and Townsend.[2]

If you find it hard to say this little word, start off slowly. Take it case by case and learn to be honest about your feelings. Don't let yourself say yes when you really want to say no. This is not fair to anyone, and over time, resentment and bitterness will build up inside of you until one day you get angry and explode. Practice *saying what you mean and meaning what you say.*

Warning: if you spend more time thinking about your to-do list than you spend living in the moment, you are overcommitted! Other people may notice that you're not much fun to be around, but the problem goes much deeper than irritability. It can affect your health. If you are already to this point, then I encourage you to set more definitive boundaries today! You are on the brink of burnout. Pick up my book *A Healthier, Happier You: 101 Steps for Lessening Stress.*[3] Remember, you can't be anything for anyone when you burn out. In fact, avoiding burnout so you can continue serving others might be *your* motivation—your "why."

I have just presented you with several tools to help you achieve good health. But it is important to remember that none of them will work unless you know your "why." Your *why* might be geared toward others, or it might be geared toward yourself.

One class member from my seasoned veteran group has arthritis. When she sticks to her workout schedule, she is able to move with minimal pain. When she doesn't make it to class, however, she feels stiff, sore, and has more pain. She is motivated and committed and knows why. Why do you want good health?

Ready for action!

Let's review what you've learned in this chapter. First, you have determined your specific health goals (SMART goals). Second, you have outlined the resources, time, and people (RTP) you need to accomplish your goal. And, last but not least, you know without a doubt *why* you are embarking on this journey.

You're ready to jump in!

FIT

Section Two

The Truth Is Out There!

50

Chapter Three

The Truth About Aging

Mark Twain once said, "I am pushing sixty. That is enough exercise for me." We laugh, but the reality is that even as we age we need to exercise. In fact, the older we get the more critical it becomes for us to exercise. Researchers are finding that inactivity, not aging, is actually the culprit behind chronic conditions such as heart disease, obesity, and osteoporosis.[1]

Your weight may stay the same over the years, but if you are not exercising, more of your body is turning to fat, according to Miriam Nelson, director of the Center for Physical Activity and Nutrition at the School of Nutrition Science and Policy at Tufts University in Boston. The good news is that it is never too late. In fact, the benefits of physical activity (cardiovascular exercise) are the same for you as they are for someone in his or her twenties: increased muscle strength, increased heart health, greater flexibility, greater endurance, more energy, and better balance. In addition, strength training (resistance training or weight training) can reverse the process of weakening muscles. A 1990 study of ten nursing home residents aged eighty-six to ninety-six had their strength boosted by an incredible 175 percent after just eight weeks of resistance training.[2]

Inactivity is a vicious cycle. The less you do, the weaker you get. Strong muscles are needed for everyday life: walking up and down stairs, carrying groceries, reaching things on high shelves, bending to pick up things, mowing grass, cleaning, and the like. The weaker you and your muscles become, the more dependent you will be. No one wants to be a burden on one's family, but not taking care of yourself could lead to a frustrating existence for all. The old saying remains true: use it or lose it. You have the choice.

Inactivity is a vicious cycle.

This chapter is going to help you distinguish between fact and fiction. What is really part of the aging process, and what is a side effect of your current lifestyle? What is normal, and what is not normal? I believe the key to aging gracefully and creating a healthy, long life is in knowing what to expect, what to accept, and what to change. Let's find the truth about the aging process once and for all.

YOU DON'T HAVE TO SUFFER

Seasoned veterans have gone through many transitions. People I know and love have gotten older: parents, friends, and class participants. I am getting older, too. We all are. We don't wake up "old" one day, although it does seem to catch up with us in our sixties.

Daniel J. Levinson states in his book *The Seasons of a Man's Life* that our lives have two halves. He claims that the second half actually begins at age forty. Up until one's forties, a person is focused on the pursuit of "things." Around forty, we have become more comfortable with who we are and what we have acquired. As we get older, we have more time to reflect, ponder, and self-evaluate. We begin to realize what is important, but we also begin to regret things done or not done.[3]

It is during this second half of life that our body begins to give out on us. These physical changes are very real reminders that we will eventually die. Seasoned veterans suffer the loss of dear friends and loved ones who begin to pass away. This increasing awareness of death and serious illness begins to affect the mind and emotions.

Our minds can remember activities we did in our childhood as if they were yesterday, but our bodies may have forgotten. Customs, traditions, and societal norms may have changed in front of our very eyes. If we are not careful, these mental and emotional changes can become discouraging. Some schools of thought even propose that depression is "par for the course" with aging. Depression is definitely higher among those over the age of fifty. The National Mental Health Association (NMHA) reports that 15 percent of adults over the age of sixty-five are affected by it. As a result, the NMHA reported that older people accept depression as part of the aging process.[4]

This is a myth. Just because we become older doesn't mean our lives are ruined, and it certainly doesn't mean that it is now acceptable to suffer. According to Lea Ann Browning McNee, senior vice president at the NMHA, "No one has to live with depression." It is this very thing that can prevent those over the age of fifty from enjoying an active and healthy life. Thus the vicious cycle: depression leads to inactivity, inactivity leads to poor quality of life, and poor quality of life leads to depression.

Change your mind today about depression. It is *not* a normal part of getting older, nor is it a sign of being weak. Depression affects millions every year, but hope exists.

It's never too late

Words have power. Say that you cannot do something, and you are likely never to do it. Ever hear people say that they feel all washed up, as if they have nothing left to give to the world? Have you ever felt as if you're just too old to matter? Thoughts such as these lead us down a very dark and lonely path.

No matter our age we all must keep a positive outlook on life. God has beautifully created us, and He has a wonderful plan for each of us. Have doubts? Check out the ages of these amazing people when they accomplished great things:[5]

- At age sixty, playwright George Bernard Shaw completed his literary masterpiece *Heartbreak House*.

- At age sixty-six, Noah Webster completed his monumental *American Dictionary of the English Language*.

- At age seventy-five, Benjamin Franklin helped draft the Declaration of Independence.

- At age eighty, Jessica Tandy became the oldest Oscar recipient for her role in *Driving Miss Daisy*. (If you haven't seen it, you must.)

- At age ninety, Pablo Picasso was still producing drawings and engravings.

- At age 102-plus, Alice Porlock of Great Britain published her first book, *Portrait of My Victory*.

- At age 119, Jeanne Calment was recognized as the oldest living person in her time.

So enough of saying, "I'm too old for that!" Yes, you are getting older, but your attitude can make all the difference in the world. And you still have much to give to this world. Don't let depression steal your joy and healthy life away.

Real issues need real help

But when do you need to get help? You may already be depressed and wonder how you can get out of "the black hole." If you experience five or more of the following symptoms for more than two weeks, seek the help of a counselor:[6]

- Persistent sad, anxious, or "empty" mood
- Sleeping too little or sleeping too much
- Change in appetite and/or weight (whether increased or decreased)
- Loss of interest in activities once enjoyed
- Restlessness, irritability
- Persistent physical symptoms that don't respond to treatment (headaches, chronic pain, or digestive disorders)

- Difficulty concentrating, remembering, or making decisions
- Fatigue or loss of energy
- Thoughts of suicide or death

Remember, depression is not something to be ashamed of. The good news is that it is treatable. A better life awaits you on the other side of depression.

AGING FACTS

If depression is not a natural part of aging, then what is? After the age of thirty-five we can expect to lose about a third of a pound of muscle each year and gain at least that much in fat, according to Miriam Nelson, director of the Center of Physical Activity.[7] Some of us will experience joint swelling and pain from years of use while others will be affected by osteoporosis. These are not a given, however. Resistance training, which creates muscle strength, also builds bone density. The healthier your bones, the less likely you will be to encounter joint swelling, pain, or osteoporosis.

Both men and women experience a decrease in hormones.

Both men and women experience a decrease in hormones starting in their thirties. Did you know that men lose 10 percent of their testosterone each year starting in their thirties? Women are not the only ones going through adjustments. Men can experience night sweats, too. Unfortunately, society has not given the same thought and consideration to the male population as they have women.[8] Women have medical help and emotional support for their transitions. Men are often unaware of their changes and left without much guidance on how to traverse the changing seas.

We can count on more changes as well. Our eyes will slowly lose their ability to focus, requiring us to use prescription glasses to read that really small print. Make it a habit to get your eyes checked at least once a year—twice a year if you have worn glasses for most of your life—to watch for signs of glaucoma and other eye problems that occur more frequently as we age.

We can also expect our hearing to decrease, but that does not mean we will all go deaf. If you have taken good care of your ears (limiting loud noises), you should not require any severe treatments. Some folks may require hearing aids, but thankfully these devices have come a long way. They are not as noticeable now, and they provide excellent amplification to live a normal life.

If you don't use it, you'll lose it.

With age comes a greater chance of stroke, heart disease, cancer, and other chronic illnesses. But remember, most of these are influenced by the choices *you* make and the life *you* live. By that I mean exercise and proper nutrition can minimize your chances of experiencing these health problems. Getting older does not equal poor quality of life. Sitting in doctor's offices each and every day and visiting the pharmacy do not have to be your future.

Use it or lose it

Our brains consist of 75 percent water. Years of not being hydrated can catch up with us, and we lose brain cells, resulting in loss of memory and senility diseases. Research is being conducted that ties Alzheimer's to long-term dehydration.[9] This is yet another incentive to drink plenty of water. We must avoid electrical waves and chemicals and limit caffeine consumption—all of which negatively impact our brain waves.

Does getting older mean we will lose our minds? No! We have better chances of keeping our wit and sharpness than we do anything else. Just remember, "If you don't use it, you'll lose it." Even our skin changes and shows the wear and tear of our life. Every wrinkle, they say, tells a story of our life. What do you want *your* story to be?

WHAT TO ACCEPT

We have all been sick at one time or another, no matter our age. But it does seem that the older we get, the more aches and pains we experience. I know about a man who is nearing fifty and feels as though his body is falling apart on him. He has shoulder soreness from years of playing tennis; he has knee pain from an old soccer injury; he has elbow pain from computer work; and he has a pulled calf from who knows what!

Some days, we can certainly feel "old" and wish we could trade in our old model for a new one. I encourage you to not give up hope. Chances are you have just gotten used to your body, worn it in like a good pair of shoes, and gotten comfortable. No, do not trade in your body; the model you have is just fine! Remember, it's all about attitude, and it's up to you.

IT'S UP TO YOU

One thing I have learned, the older I have got,
In how we approach life, our attitude means a lot.

We will get older and face difficult days.
People will hurt us with their actions and with what
they say.

We will lose things and loved ones we hold dear.
Aches, pains, and illness may appear.

Our financial situation could get tough.
At times, we might feel like we have had enough.

It is then that we have power that we cannot see.
It is the realization that "I can only work on me."

You can't change the past or what you have done.
You can only believe, trust, and lean on the One.

What really matters is what you think in your head.
It isn't so much what happens to you, but what is said.

Your words and attitude toward a situation are paramount.
It is what truly counts.

Your attitude is what will get you through
And keep you "pressing on" even when you are blue.

Positive thinking can overcome the biggest mountaintop
Or negative thinking can create the world's worst flop.

Choose to change how you look at life
And you will reduce stress, illness, and strife.

Talk positively and see things turn around.
May He keep you in His care so that you will abound!

—LORRAINE BOSSÉ-SMITH

We can certainly take measures to improve our health and reduce our chances of disease, but some things will just happen as part of the natural course of aging. You do need to accept the fact that you are getting older.

Being sick is expensive.

However, your attitude is one of the most important tools you have for combating depression and disease. Constantly put things in perspective. For example, maybe you don't like wearing glasses, but it sure beats being blind. Every day I wake up is a good day. We are so incredibly blessed to be alive. When things go wrong, a positive attitude can get you through to the other side quickly. Never underestimate the power you have within you. God gives us hope. It is a gift; let us not waste it.

Pay now or pay later

We all know that it is not cheap to treat ailments, illness, and disease. The Society for Women's Health recently decided to determine how expensive it is. They found that it would run a woman about $423,000 over her lifetime to treat cardiovascular disease. This includes high blood pressure and obesity. This is *her* cost, not her insurance company's. Diabetes will cost approximately $233,000. Urinary incontinence is $58,000.[10]

To the average person, these figures are alarming. What they tell me is that we will either pay today with our effort and time exercising, or we will pay later with our wallets. The choice is ours.

What to Change

So what should you change? As I mentioned before, we can do something about 70 percent of the process.

I believe that exercise is the key to maintaining a healthy life well into our maturity. And as I stated before, we *can* do something about our health—starting today. Exercise can increase your longevity, improve your quality of life, and increase your mobility and independence. Here are some immediate changes you can make today:

- Eat a lot of fruits and vegetables.

- Avoid fatty/fried foods.

- Limit your dairy intake (use rice or soy milk or low-fat cow's milk).

- Exercise your body at least three times a week (to help heart, muscles, bone density, and mental alertness).

- Stretch every day (to maintain flexibility).

- Get the right amount of sleep—not too little or too much. (Our muscles can recover with a short break, but our brains cells can be restored only with sleep.)

- Exercise your brain every day (crossword puzzles, word games, multitasking, Bible verse memorization).

- Build a strong social network of friends and peers.

- Drink plenty of water (to help skin, brain cells, muscles, organs, and overall health).

Work within your level

One thing I have worked really hard at during my seasoned veteran fitness classes is to not focus on what participants cannot do. My theory has been that every morning they wake up, they know *exactly* what they cannot do. What they'd rather focus on is what they *can* do. I call it "working within your level."

Besides what we do or don't do, we all have genes that predetermine some level of health. Why is it that some people can run their entire lives and never have a knee injury while someone else's knees blow out in their thirties? Genetics. I will not go very deep into this subject, but knowing your family genes can help you understand potential trouble areas so that you can focus your efforts on avoiding them.

Work within your ability.

My siblings and I have a longstanding joke that we really don't know what runs in our family because everyone died of cancer by the age of fifty-five. We don't know if heart disease or diabetes is in our genes—only time will tell. What we have learned is that cancer is prevalent. What have I done about it? I have avoided alcohol and smoking and have exercised and eaten a healthy diet my entire life. I try to manage my stress day by day, and I pray for good health. But still, we alone can only do so much. We need a greater power.

LEANING ON GOD

That leads me to the last-but-not-least thing you can do to stay young and healthy. Every one of us has faced or will face a time in our lives when things do not go well, despite our best efforts. It is during these times that we have to lean upon God and trust in His grace and mercy. God loves us and is right beside us. I hope you know that and believe it with all your heart. On those days that you are feeling alone, isolated, and perhaps even useless to this world, please know that you are loved very much. You are valuable and have great worth. God knows you by name, and He knows your circumstances.

Prayer always changes me.

I have found great comfort in the words of C. S. Lewis: "Prayer does not always change my circumstances, but it always changes me." Prayer and meditation can help you stay focused on what is truly important. As you take steps toward a healthy life, never forget to look up at the One who made you. With Him, all things are possible.

Chapter Four

The Truth About
Cardiovascular Exercise

Our world is not lacking in information. Some people call this the Information Age. I call it the Overload Age. In this day you can obtain just about any piece of information you want or need through a variety of sources: newspaper, magazines, television, library, the Internet, and so on. We cannot seem to get away from information. We have computers, cell phones, telephones, pagers, fax machines, and televisions bombarding us every day.

Mark Sanborn is a national speaker who tells the story of the day he was at the airport using his cell phone to check his voice mail. He inadvertently dialed his own cell phone number, and as his cell phone rang, he answered it. He heard this man saying, "Hello? Who is this?" It took him a few minutes to discover he was talking to himself. Now that's what I call information overload! What are we to do with all of this information, and how do we sort it out?

It is very frustrating for most people, especially when it comes to health and fitness, to find the truth. What *is* the right thing to do, and whom do you trust? I hope by now you know that my desire is simply to help you get healthy. I am not selling you anything or pushing a fad on you. I am simply taking some time-tested, scientifically proven theories and bringing them down to a practical level. I really am here to help. But all of the information I give you will not do anything for you. You must apply the information to your life.

My goal is to motivate you toward a healthier life, keep you safe while you do it, and encourage you to stay with it for the rest of your life. I do not want to overwhelm you with too many details. If, however, you would like to gain a more in-depth knowledge of health and fitness, I suggest *Fitness and Health* by Brian J. Sharkey, PhD.[1] Although Sharkey does not focus the book on those over the age of fifty, he does address the aging process. You might also go onto the Internet and check www.agingresearch.org for more articles on health for seasoned veterans.

This chapter covers the basics of fitness and health. It's what every seasoned veteran should know.

Healthy Hearts

Staying healthy requires us to address three aspects of our health: cardiovascular capacity (heart health), muscle strength and endurance (for healthy bones), and flexibility (mobility). In this chapter, we will discuss your cardiovascular capacity, which is simply your ability to take in oxygen and process it, which is why cardio exercise is so important. *USA Today,* in their August 23, 2004 edition, reported that the number of women with high blood pressure has caught up to the number of men, putting women at a higher risk for heart disease.

To illustrate the growing need for improved cardio health, let me describe a scenario I see happening all the time. Our church sits on top of a hill. If you park at the lower lot, you must walk up a flight of stairs. I have been constantly amazed at how many people get completely out of breath taking those few steps, and when they finally get to the top, they can hardly breathe. Many of them take the entire church service to catch their breath. This is dangerous! Their hearts are in very bad shape, and oxygen is not getting where it is needed. This puts those folks at a higher risk for disease.

Did you know that there is a direct correlation between being overweight and diabetes and coronary heart disease? In other words, managing one's weight can reduce the likelihood of these diseases—at any age!

What happens when you try to clean the house with a vacuum cleaner whose bag is already full? When a vacuum cleaner has no place to put the incoming dirt and dust, it starts to kick it back out. Over time, it becomes completely clogged and stops working altogether. A vacuum cleaner's maintenance is pretty easy. All you have to do is change the bag on a regular basis and check the belt. A little attention keeps all the mobile parts working properly.

In the same way, if you don't maintain your heart, it will get clogged. If mistreated, it will cause all sorts of problems. And if it is ignored for a long period of time, it may stop running altogether.

We can't expect our vacuum cleaners to run perfectly if we haven't changed the bags, so how can we expect our hearts to function when we haven't been kind to them? Be kind to your heart! Do what it takes to keep it healthy!

Cardiovascular exercise can dramatically reduce your chances of age-related diseases. Let me explain how.

Benefits of a healthy heart

The greater the workload on your heart, the more efficient it needs to become. When you become completely winded from an easy endeavor, like the people walking up a flight of stairs at church, it means your cardio capacity is not very good. Your body is not producing enough oxygen for the required work. But the greater your capacity to process oxygen and use it, the lower your blood pressure will be because the heart does not have to work as hard to get what it needs.

Your goal is to get your heart operating more efficiently. When your heart is weak, it has to work harder to produce enough oxygen to support your body, and this raises your blood pressure. Standards for blood pressure have recently been lowered because of the known association with heart disease. Don't let a lack of cardiovascular exercise put you at risk.

Cardio exercise will not only reduce your chances of heart disease, but it will also help with your circulation. Oxygen helps blood get to all parts of your body. The stronger your heart, the better your blood will flow, which will eliminate most circulation problems. If you presently struggle with poor circulation, look at increasing your cardiovascular exercise.

Many people take medicines that may not be necessary. Exercise and a well-balanced diet can sometimes do the trick! I am angry at all the commercials on television these days selling drugs. On one hand, we have the fight against drugs, yet on the other, we are encouraging folks to take them. I am not against medicine, which has allowed us all to live better lives. But I am against taking medications for problems we have created and can solve through exercise and nutrition.

Changing metabolism

The older you become the more difficulty you may have losing weight. I will not lie and tell you that you can lose weight as easily as people who are in their thirties, but you *can* lose it. Your body's metabolism has changed and will continue to change as you age. No one is immune to this. Growing older means the body's metabolism is slowing down. But it is still working. It will just require paying attention to what goes in and how you work it off more than you have in the past.

WAIST-TO-HIP RATIO

Let's pause for a moment right now and see how you're doing. Get a tape measure and take your waist and hip measurements. Divide your waist measurement by your hip measurement. The result is your waist-to-hip ratio.

> Waist measurement = _____ (WM)
> Hip measurement = _____ (HM)
> WM ____ divided by HM ____ = ____ (waist-to-hip ratio)[2]

For example, if your waist measures 36 inches and your hips measure 43 inches, your waist-to-hip ratio would be .84. If your waist is at 50 inches and your hips are at 44 inches, your waist-to-hip ratio would be 1.14. The lower the number the better.

Men with a ratio higher than .95 and women with a ratio greater than .85 are in the high-fat category and have a greater risk for heart attack. If you fall into this category, you need to lose weight as soon as possible.[3] For a more comprehensive diagnosis, I encourage you to visit your physician. Your doctor can assess your body fat. The higher the fat content in your body, the higher your risk for heart disease and other ailments.

Even if your measurements are acceptable—meaning they are lower than the numbers I just mentioned—you must continually include cardio exercise in your routine in order to prevent future health problems. Remember, you want to live a long and *healthy* life. What good is living to 100 if you can't do the things you enjoy?

Note that there is a big difference between being thin and being healthy. I have seen many skinny seasoned veterans who eat like birds and do not exercise. If you are in this category, please know that you are in danger. You can be thin and still have an unhealthy heart, weak muscles, and frail bones. If you were to fall, you could break something because you lack the muscle mass that not only increases bone density but also protects the bone from fractures.

Daily decisions

A friend of mine who is in his mid-fifties now does not allow one impure thing to touch his lips. In his twenties and thirties, however, he ate pretty much anything he wanted. He just made sure he worked out hard. When he got to his forties, he began slowly removing some unhealthy items from his diet, and then when he hit his fifties he felt it was time to get "serious." He doesn't feel deprived, because he lived it up when he was young. What he is doing now is ensuring that he has many more good years ahead, and that is more important than eating whatever he wants.

I'm not suggesting you go this extreme, but I wanted to illustrate the point that some adjustments will need to be made. It will be worth the small sacrifice, though.

Working out right

If I had to guess, I would say that over 90 percent of the people who come to me desiring to lose weight are not exercising hard enough. This is frustrating for them, because they're working out but not seeing the results they want. Some of these people are dedicating an entire hour to cardiovascular exercise every day, but they are working at such a slow pace that they are not getting the health benefit. How discouraging!

Cardio exercise improves your circulation.

As a fitness professional I want to help folks know more about exercising so they can receive the benefits. Why put in the workout time if you're not doing it right or getting any improvements to your health?

The Aerobics and Fitness Association of America (AFAA) has found that 80 percent of Americans do not get enough of the right level of exercise on a weekly basis to receive any health benefit. That means only 20 percent of Americans are exercising correctly, even though a lot more people are at the gym.[4] Never fear. You are about to learn a very simple, customized approach to determining if you are working out at the right intensity level.

How Hard Should I Work Out?

Below is a chart I have fine-tuned from something called the rate of perceived exertion (RPE).[5] It's a way of tracking your workout intensity level based on how hard you're breathing. This will help you understand the levels of intensity you may reach as you're working out. Just remember to monitor *your* breathing and no one else's. You are working out for you and your health.

Chart 4.1—Workout Intensity Chart

Intensity	Description
1	Very light exercise—breathing through nose, easy to talk. *Usually seated activities*
2	Light exercise—breathing fuller through nose with deeper breaths. *Gardening, walking the dog*
3	Slightly moderate exercise—breathing pattern begins to change, deeper and less controlled. *Fast walking, shoveling snow or dirt*
4	Moderate exercise—breathing through mouth begins. You can still speak, but not quite as easily. *Taking the stairs, leisurely riding a bike*
5	Strong exercise—labored but controlled breathing through the mouth; more difficult to talk now. *Jogging, cycling long distance*
6	Hard exercise—labored but controlled breathing; you must now take a breath every few words to maintain a conversation. *Exercise class (end of warm-up), swimming*
7	Very hard exercise—labored, heavier breathing through mouth; "comfortably uncomfortable." *Exercise class (mid-way through class), playing tennis or basketball*
8	Very, very hard exercise—labored, heavier breathing; "uncomfortable but doable." Talking is very limited and difficult. *Exercise class (visit level 8 during class), jumping rope, or elliptical*
9	Extremely hard exercise—begin breathless stage; talking is extremely difficult. *Exercise class (only a few minutes of class at this level), running*
10	Maximum effort—complete breathlessness; no talking at all.

This chart works because it is it is completely customizable to your age, gender, and physical shape. Level 6 for you will not be the same as for the next person—so it works for everyone. It also takes into account how you are feeling that particular day as well as what you have eaten and what prescriptions you have taken. You might be fighting a cold or struggling with allergies. Some days you may just feel "tired." On those days you need to adjust your level accordingly. (In chapter ten I provide you with a journal that records how you are feeling. Use this to help with your exercise selection for the day.) When your body is not as strong, do something lighter. Other days you might be feeling fine and can increase your intensity and challenge your cardio capacity. We are not machines. Do your best every day.

I have had several clients come to me recently who were stuck at a weight they didn't like. On the surface, it appeared they were doing the right things. One gal was running on her treadmill for a full hour each day, and another was cycling on her stationary bike in her home several times a week for thirty minutes at a time. But they weren't losing any weight, which had left them very frustrated.

I asked some key questions about their intensity. The gal on the treadmill was going at a snail's pace, and the other was reading really good books that required a lot of thought while she cycled. Neither of these gals was working out hard enough. It didn't take me long to discover the key to their success was increasing their intensity. They needed to breathe hard enough to work their hearts, thereby burning calories and fat. These girls, as well as other clients of mine, have adjusted their workouts and have seen results immediately. One gal lost several inches in a matter of weeks, and the other lost almost twenty pounds.

NOTE: When exercising outside, remember to consider the heat index. As I write this book we have had a severe heat wave with high humidity. Advisories have been posted warning people not to overexert themselves and to drink plenty of liquids. Take this into account. And don't forget elevation, either. If you are not accustomed to higher altitudes but travel to places such as Colorado, adjust your intensity when you work out at those higher elevations. You will find your body working harder simply because of the heat or lower amounts of oxygen in the air.

Here's a rule of thumb: if you can say "supercalifragilisticexpialidocious" in one breath while you are exercising, you're not working hard enough. You need to increase your intensity. When you are working at the right level, you will need to take a breath while saying that very long word. In addition, if you can work out while reading a book or magazine without feeling sick, you are not working hard enough either (sorry, multitaskers).

How Often Should I Work Out?

I believe in "cumulative exercise," which means that you can count everyday activities toward your total exercise goal. Don't underestimate what you do: yard work, housework, washing cars, and taking the stairs add up.

But remember, the body is designed to move. The heart needs to be challenged in order to remain strong. Certainly, getting out and moving is good for you, but if you truly want to improve your cardio capacity and reduce your chances of heart disease, then you must work the body hard enough.

My training clients often ask me how often they should work out. We all have different goals, so the specific answer varies. However, the Aerobics and Fitness Association of America (AFAA, from whom I received my certifications and credentials) recommends exercising three to five times a week. Research has proven that this frequency will maintain your level of health.

As a fifty-plus individual, this is a perfect goal for your cardio exercise. If you can find an exercise class that also incorporates some body sculpting or resistance training, then you have everything you need.

You may have to build up to three times a week, but don't give up. Remember that daily activities count. Be creative, too. Try different things, and do what you love. This is often a perfect place to start.

Tim, one of my fifty-plus class members, loves to play doubles tennis with the guys. They are out there several times a week playing tournaments. He makes sure he gets his three aerobic classes in at the gym, but then he plays tennis throughout the week for fun—and extra exercise. For Tim it's also a social outlet, time to shoot the breeze with friends. Tim used to smoke and was overweight. Today he is in better shape in his sixties than he was in his thirties. (Tim is one of the models for this book.) Our bodies are amazing and will respond if we just do the right things. Remember, it's never too late!

If you desire to lose some weight, then research suggests that you must exercise more than three days a week. Try adding another day or two to your schedule as Tim does. Again, be creative and find things you enjoy. Regardless of your goal, don't forget to plan exercise into your weekly schedule: walking the dog, talking a stroll along the beach, gardening, and the like. The bottom line here is to ensure you are exercising enough times throughout the week to improve your heart's ability.

Work out safely

Now I will make a special note. You should really receive your doctor's clearance before embarking on any new fitness or exercise regimen. Please do not take this lightly. You are exercising to *improve* your health, not damage it. You don't need an injury or trauma to set you back. It's not worth it.

Don't buy into the saying "no pain; no gain." Nothing could be further from the truth. As we get older, it will take less for our heart rates to climb. Monitor your heart rate and breathing closely. If you start to feel lightheaded or dizzy, STOP immediately. If, however, you are simply out of breath and need to catch it, adjust your intensity briefly.

A friend of mine is really good at this. She will run at a high intensity until she needs a quick break, then she will walk for only a few steps—just long enough to get her breath—and then she goes back to running. She is sixty! This is called *interval training* and is an awesome way to receive health benefits. Varying your intensity is fine. You just need to make sure that you get your total time in at that proper level.

Any time your arms are up over your head, your heart rate will be higher. Lower your arms to lower your heart rate. If you are moving around, walk in place instead. When running, take smaller strides to ease the intensity a bit. These are all ways to keep working out safely and effectively. Use the Workout Intensity Chart to ensure you are working out properly but safely.

How Long Should I Work Out?

Gone are the days of exercising just twenty minutes a few times a week. Because of the sedentary lives we live, we need more exercise today than in years past. Some agencies strongly advise one hour a day every day, while others suggest thirty minutes a day, three to five days a week.

I'm a realist. I love to exercise, but one hour *every day* is nearly impossible when you have other commitments. Be flexible. We can all get in a few days of exercise in a week...maybe not all in one-hour increments. Don't be so rigid with your workout that you don't allow life to happen. But do get at least thirty minutes of cardio exercise in your schedule several times a week.

If you can afford a full hour of exercise on your workout days (such as attending a class), then you are doing great. Any additional times you add are bonuses! Of course, if you do need to lose weight, you must exercise more often to get to a healthy weight. Afterwards you can maintain with a reduced schedule. Just remember to do it! The best plans unrealized are way worse than the "OK" plan executed today.

To work out or not to work out...that is the question

Another question I am often asked by clients is whether they should work out if they are sick. Here's a guideline for you to follow: if you do not have a fever, then go ahead and work out, but adjust your intensity. Sweating actually helps your body release toxins more quickly, even when you are sick. If, however, you are running a temperature, do not exercise. Your body is fighting the sickness, and it needs all its strength to recover from the illness.

Missing a day or two won't hurt you, but exercising with a fever can put you in bed for weeks! Listen to your body. You have lived with it for many years, and listening to what it is telling you beats any advice I can give you. I like to say, "Listen to your body's whisper today or hear it scream tomorrow."

I made the mistake recently of thinking, *One time won't hurt me.* I was running a fever from the nasty flu bug going around, which I normally can kick out of my system quickly. But I decided to teach a fitness class anyway. I worked at full capacity and taxed my body so much that I got the full-blown bug. Yuck! I was sick for three weeks instead of my typical couple of days. This rule can't be broken, not even once.

Prescription drug alert

Many seasoned veterans are or will be on some sort of medication. I am not opposed to medications, especially when they can improve our health. As I mentioned earlier, I just do not agree with them when we can do something about our condition without them (such as losing weight and trimming down). But if you are on a medication (or two or more), please check with your doctor or pharmacist to learn how it will impact your exercise. (The journal in chapter ten will give you a place to record what you have taken for the day.) Some medications will increase your heart rate, so you will have to adapt your exercise accordingly. Others will keep it low, so you have to carefully watch your breathing. Learn as much as you can about the drugs you are taking and their side effects. It is good to be in the know.

Sample intensity change

Below is a typical fifty-plus aerobics (low impact/sculpting) class format so that you can begin to see how hard you should be working and when:

- Warm-up—usually ten minutes. Intensity is low, level one to four. You are breathing through your nose, but by the end of warm-up you are feeling warm and are taking fuller breaths.

- Low impact—about twenty minutes. The core of the cardiovascular exercise comes next with medium intensity, ranging from level five to seven on the workout intensity chart. You are raising your arms up, moving quicker and breathing harder. You can talk but sporadically and not in complete sentences.

- High impact—five minutes. For those who feel they are able to push it, I lead my classes into a brief period that challenges them to "visit" the higher intensity levels (eight through ten), but only momentarily. You should not push to the point of dizziness. You will, however, feel breathless…like you can't do this for long. And you won't. You will have your legs higher up and cover more ground, moving even quicker.

- Sculpting—While your core body temperature is warmer and your muscles are engaged, most classes will introduce the resistance training part of the class (usually around twenty minutes). Working the muscles right after your cardio exercise will help your body burn a few extra calories! Light weights and exercise bands are often used. While your heart rate is still up, do not bend over or immediately go to the floor. Stay upright until you have a chance to catch your breath.

- Floor work—five to eight minutes. After some weight-bearing exercise, you may be asked to weave in some sit-ups and other floor work designed to build core strength. These are awesome for any age.

- Cool down—The last five to eight minutes of your class should be cool down and stretch. Your heart rate should have slowly begun to come down from the highest point. Remember that as one gets older, there are changes in the ability to recover. It may take a little longer for your heart rate to come back down, but if you do the right things you should feel good at the end of your workout. By the end of cool down you want your heart rate in the lower intensity range: one to four. You should be able to breathe through your nose comfortably again. Never just stop without a cool down period. Always take time to stretch out the muscles that you used during the workout.

If you don't attend a class designed for fifty-plus individuals, you can follow this same approach with your own workout. Start off low, work the longest portion at the medium intensity level, visit the high level briefly, then cool down.

CARDIOVASCULAR TEST

You will want to monitor your progress, in order for you to see improvements. You must, therefore, know where you started. I would like you to take a five-minute cardiovascular test that will give you an indication of your "heart fitness level." You will need a step or low stool, a watch, a piece of paper, and a pencil. Here's how it goes:

1. Take your heart rate by putting two fingers on your radial pulse (wrist). Once you find it, count the beats you feel in a ten-second span.

2. Record this number on a sheet of paper.

3. Then for five minutes, step up and down, leading with your right leg then left. Maintain a relatively good pace—not super slow but not a mad dash.

4. At the end of your five minutes, sit down and take your pulse again for ten seconds.

5. Record this number, and make note of how hard you're breathing.

6. Mark down what intensity level you feel you achieved based on the chart I outlined.

7. Continue to sit down for five minutes, breathing normally.

8. After five minutes, take your pulse one more time for ten seconds.

9. Record this number, and note your breathing.

How high did your second pulse number get as compared to the first? If it is more than twenty beats, you need to improve your cardiovascular health, especially if your third number did not come back down to the first number. Remember, the healthier your heart is, the quicker it will recover. You should get very close to your original number and breathing pattern after resting for five minutes. Use this as your benchmark, and see the results unfold as you commit to exercising on a regular basis.

Easy does it

One more caution: pace yourself. Don't try to fix years of an unhealthy lifestyle in two weeks! Take it slow, but make it meaningful. Remember that small steps *will* make a difference.

Small steps get you there.

Chapters six, seven, and eight will help you begin to make those steps based on your stage in life. Cardiovascular exercises, strength training, and stretching will be outlined for you with pictures and helpful tips. Find the ones that fit you, your lifestyle, and your goals. Remember that small steps get you there.

Chapter Five

The Truth About Weight-Bearing Exercise

So far our quest for truth has helped us understand the aging process: what we can expect and what we can change. I hope you were encouraged and inspired to take charge of your future. The quality of your health will be dramatically influenced by what you choose to do and not do. Our search for the truth has also informed us on the proper way of exercising our heart so that we get the health benefit. If we are going to put the time in, let's get something out of it!

Our journey now takes us to weight-bearing exercise, something misunderstood by many people, young and old alike. It is a critical part of the equation and should not be ignored.

A gal I know, who is only in her late forties, had not exercised much during her life. Recently, she fell off her 4 x 4 motorbike and broke her wrist in several places. Her doctor said that if she had more muscles, she would have sprained it, not broken it. In other words, she didn't have enough muscle mass to protect the bones and the bones were weak. In my family, our ankles are weak. But I have worked on strengthening my ankles so that, unlike others, I can twist my ankle and walk it off. I have built up muscle strength and bone density. The two are related, but I didn't always know that.

WHY WEIGHT-BEARING EXERCISE?

For a long time I was one of the many people who didn't like to lift weights—so I didn't. Most women don't like it. Some fear, as I did, that they will grow big, ugly, masculine muscles. I simply wanted to stay lean and trim. I finally learned that weight-bearing exercise will help do just that. Here's the truth:

The stronger your muscles, the healthier your bones!

Try this exercise: raise your arms straight out in front of you (as if you were sleepwalking). How hard is this to hold? It shouldn't be very hard. After a while, it would get tiring, but not painful. Now, if you had your arms out in front of you, but I began pushing down on them with all my weight, how long could you sustain that position without lowering them? You have my resistance working against you.

It is this very resistance that your muscles and bones require to stay healthy. Moving your arms and legs isn't working out; it is ordinary movement. But add resistance that forces the muscles to contract and pull against the bone, and you have *workload*.

Workload is the force that makes your muscles pull against the bones. Bones that experience this force become denser and stronger, because they have to in order to sustain the force against them. Bones with little or no resistance, on the contrary, have no need to grow big and strong—that is where osteoporosis comes in. It is just the opposite of strong and healthy bones. If you have been diagnosed with osteoporosis, then resistance training is a mandatory activity for you.

A friend of mine was diagnosed with osteoporosis in her twenties. She was losing bone density at a rapid pace until she met me. We discussed the importance of weight-bearing exercise and added it to her weekly routine. She has regained strength and density. Recently, she fell off her mammoth donkey, breaking her elbow. She began to heal so quickly that the doctors didn't put her in a cast. And in a month's time, she was healed—a far cry from what her bones were like when she was in her twenties!

Our bodies are amazing. Changing your habits today can still make a positive impact on your future. And it is never too late. Even if you have been struggling with osteoporosis, you can make improvements with resistance training.

Adding resistance training to your regimen does not guarantee that you will never have another broken bone. But it will create denser, stronger muscles that will reduce that likelihood. When I work with seasoned veterans, I like to remind them that much of our exercise is preventative. Think of what you are doing today for the "what ifs" of tomorrow. What if you fell down the stairs? What if you did step off that curb wrong? What you are doing by exercising is creating the best scenario possible—equipping your body to take the blow. Hopefully you won't fall off a horse or big donkey, but you never know. And if you do, you want your body to be ready.

Testimony of healthy muscles and bones

I have been incorporating weight-bearing exercise in my regimen for years now. I have a healthy body fat percentage, toned muscles, and strong bones. How do I know? I found out the hard way. A couple of years ago now, I learned how to ride a motorcycle. I took the course and got my license. On a trip with some friends, I decided to take a spin on a friend's bike. My first mistake was that I did so even though I was not familiar with his bike. My second mistake was that this bike was much bigger than the one I had learned on—about double the size. My third and biggest mistake was that my protective riding gear was in my husband's bike ahead of me. But I started her up for a short little jaunt in the desert.

I thought I would be fine for just a few miles. Well, that was all it took. Not far down the road I took a turn too wide, and I hit the ground going forty miles per hour. I hit the pavement hard, landing on my left hip, left elbow, and left knee. The bike came crashing down on me, pushing me deep into the black top.

I had horrible road rash, cuts, abrasions, and deep wounds. But as serious and painful as this crash was, I did not sustain a single broken bone. After hearing about the wreck, the doctors were sure I had broken my elbow and kneecap. X-rays indicated otherwise. The only explanation the doctors could come up with was that I had strong muscles that protected my bones and that my bones were dense and thick, thus allowing them to sustain the blow. I never hurt so badly in my life, but I was also very thankful it was not worse.

Resistance training will improve your bone health.

Don't wait to find out the hard way how important it is to your health that you lift weights. Incorporate resistance training into your life now.

Just as we need cardiovascular exercise, so we must lift weights. Here are some guidelines for doing it properly.

How Often Should I Lift?

While our bodies are designed to handle cardiovascular exercise every day, our muscles need rest. They need to recover and heal.

You will want to lift weights at least one time a week for a maintenance program. Adding a second day of resistance training will ensure healthy muscles and bones. Most classes for fifty-plus individuals include resistance training in every class, three times a week. With a day of rest in between, this is fine. Often, the classes can't get to every muscle group, so they are focusing on different ones each class. Another approach is to do the upper body one day and the lower body the next. With that schedule, you could lift four days a week: two upper and two lower. If you don't enjoy giving it that much time, get all your muscles in at once or attend a class.

Are you familiar with indoor moss? I use it for my floral arrangements. It comes in brown, beige, and green. When you buy it, it is in a small, compact bag. When you open it up, you begin to pull at it and tear it apart. Before you know it, the little bag of moss is a *big* pile of moss. It got torn apart and created more moss as a result. That is what your muscles are doing when you work them—coming apart so that they can multiply. And more muscle mass is better! Muscles support your every move, so you want lots of muscle as you get older.

NOTE: The process of working out your muscles shouldn't be painful. You may have some tenderness, but with a proper cool down and stretch, you should not truly hurt. If at any time you begin to really hurt, *stop*. Pain is not the name of this game.

How Hard Should I Lift?

Lifting weights is not a race. You're not trying to get your heart rate up now, so the Workout Intensity Chart doesn't apply here. What you're striving for when you lift is good form.

What exactly *is* good form? I'm glad you asked!

Remember how I explained the force your muscles are sustaining? That is a key to lifting properly: using your muscles, not your joints. We want those muscles to pull on the bones, but that won't happen if you use your joints. The best way to avoid this is to never lock your knees or elbows when lifting. When you find yourself doing this, it may be an indication that you are trying to lift too much weight. The other important aspect of form is to slow it down. The faster you go, the less work your muscles are really performing.

It was true with cardio exercise, and it is true here: if you are going to put the time in, make it count!

Lift and lower slowly

In order to get the biggest health benefit, you want to not only lift your weights slowly, but you also want to lower them slowly. If you ever hear weights slamming down at the gym, you can be sure that people are using their joints more than their muscles, and they have momentum on their side.

You may already have some arthritis (joint swelling) from youthful injuries, and some of your joints may have pain. You don't want to add pain by lifting wrong. Rather, you want to build stronger muscles so that the joints are protected and bones are strengthened. Therefore, make your muscles work on the up and the down, the lift and the lower. The technical terms for the two phases are *concentric* and *eccentric* movements.[1] If you are interested in learning more about this, see my book *Finally FIT!*[2]

Bicep curl example

I don't want you to get too hung up on the terms. I simply want you to understand that it is more effective and safer to lift slowly. Perhaps an example will help illustrate and be more effective than definitions. Let's look at a basic bicep curl.

A bicep curl requires you to curl up a weight with your arm. You start with your arm almost straight down by your leg, but don't lock

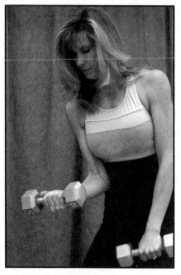

the elbow straight—keep a slight bend. As you slowly lift the weight toward you, your wrists will face your body. While you are lifting your arm (bending it), your muscle is in a *concentric* contraction, working *against* gravity. It is heavy and difficult to hold here because gravity wants to lower your arm back down. This is the hardest workload since you are "pulling," and this is where you would breathe out. (More on breathing below.) But it is just as important to maintain control when you lower the weight, going with gravity, as the weight returns to its original position (*eccentric* phase).

NOTE: It is during the concentric contraction that you should breathe out. Breathing in on the eccentric portions gets oxygen to the muscles in preparation for the workload. Breathing out on the pull helps give you power by releasing the oxygen. You can use your breathing as an excellent tool to slow you down. It will help you resist the temptation to quickly pull up or lower down.

How Long Should I Lift?

The good news here is that, unlike cardio exercise, you have options. You don't have to follow any guidelines for how much time you invest in lifting. Granted, you can't rush lifting. You must honor the lifting and lowering slowly principle, but you can work efficiently. That means you can alternate muscle groups instead of resting and get your entire body done in thirty minutes! Or you can take your breaks and work out a full hour. Your goals and schedule will determine this aspect more than anything.

A word you will hear and should become familiar with is a *rep*. This is simply how many times you lift. As in a class, if the instructor counts to ten and you lift ten, you just performed ten repetitions (reps). If she has you do the same exercise again, then you will have completed a second "set," or the number of times you do your reps consecutively. Later on in this chapter I provide suggestions for the number of reps and sets based upon your age and objectives.

You've got style!

Something I have added to resistance training is the idea of personality styles. Your personality style greatly impacts what kind of weight resistance will work best for you. (See my book *Finally FIT!* for suggestions.)

For our purposes today, I encourage you to check out either a fitness class that weaves in both cardio and resistance training so that you have a group atmosphere or a quick circuit program such as Curves. Typically, you can be in and out in thirty minutes with a circuit format. Many gyms are incorporating these into their schedule, so it is not just for women. Men lead busy lives, too!

Let's go swimming

Don't have time to go to a class? Here is a great resistance training exercise that I like to offer folks who can't afford a health or fitness club or are just plain busy. It is a routine I call "swimming."

All you need is a set of light hand weights that you can buy inexpensively. Women should start off with three-pound weights, with the goal of increasing their resistance to five or six pounds. Men should be able to easily start off at five- or six-pound weights and move to eight or ten pounds rather quickly. Don't go too heavy. Make sure you have fluid, unstrained movement. I like to play music while I do this, but it is up to you. We're going swimming!

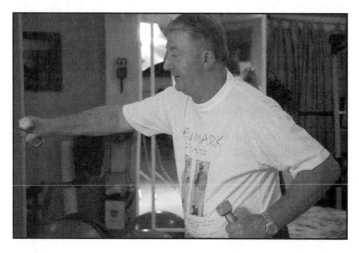

With your legs spread comfortably apart and your knees "soft," stand up nice and tall facing forward. Have one weight in each hand. Begin with moving your arms forward, one at a time, as if you are doing the doggy paddle. Right arm, then your left arm—this is one rep; continue to ten reps.

Make sure you breathe in when the weights are close to you and breathe out when they are away from you. You are working your shoulder rotation and mobility, not to mention your biceps, triceps, and deltoids.

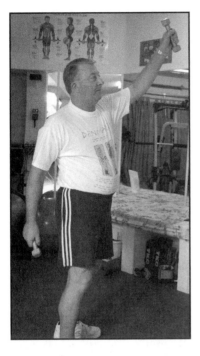

When you are finished with the doggy paddle, proceed to the backstroke (behind or backwards), one arm at a time, counting to ten again. Now you know why swimmers have great upper bodies: it is the resistance! What you are doing with the hand weights is simulating the resistance of the water on your upper body. Continue to keep your knees soft and breathe out on the push.

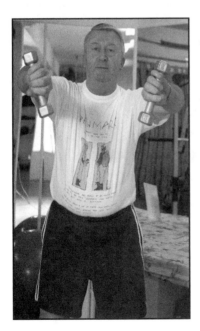

After the backstroke, move to the breaststroke. Both arms start off with the weights together in the front by your chest bone (sternum). Press both arms out in front of you, and then push them away from each other. You are literally mirroring a breaststroke in the water, but you have the hand weights instead. Count to ten, and keep breathing. Remember to keep your knees soft (slightly bent).

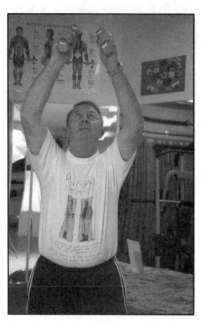

You're almost finished. The last segment is what I call the dive. You push the weights straight up over your head (shoulder press) and then bring them down to your side using the back muscles. Move your arms straight up and then straight down to your sides, just as you would in a jumping jack. Be sure that your elbows are not locked, but keep your arms relatively straight. Count to ten once more.

If you're game, repeat the entire swimming routine a second or third time. This should take only about ten to twenty minutes, depending on how many sets you do. But in this short amount of time, you will have worked your entire upper body.

When I travel, I bring hand weights with me just in case the hotel does not have a weight room. A woman from one of my workshops suggested water weights. These are empty plastic weights that you fill with water to the appropriate level or weight. When you are done, you drain them, which makes it much lighter to travel. What an idea! I recently saw them advertised in an in-flight magazine, but I am sure you can get them in any travel-equipment store.

Regardless of your age and ability, this swimming routine is an excellent way to work your entire upper body.

Pros and Cons

The different types of resistance training have their pros and cons. No option is better or worse. You must simply use whichever fits your needs, lifestyle, and goals. I like a combination! Here are some things to consider when deciding between handheld weights, free weights, and weight-lifting machines.

Handheld weights

You may have a set of these for walking. They were very popular in the 1980s. They are still an awesome way to work your muscles, because they are so easy to use. They are relatively inexpensive, and you can use them anywhere (at home, traveling, and so forth). They also require that you use your core muscles, which is an added bonus.

Free weights

Free weights are similar to handheld weights but are larger and usually involve bars and pulley devices. They are really a cross between handheld weights and weight-lifting machines. They can be more dangerous because you don't have a machine helping you or protecting you. You must stabilize yourself and the weight. These are good to weave in with proper execution up until age sixty, at which point I'd encourage you to switch to handheld weights or weight-lifting machines, unless you have years of experience with free weights and feel very comfortable with them. A workout buddy is a must with free weights.

Weight-lifting equipment

The equipment you will find at health clubs and gyms will vary in size, difficulty, effectiveness, and safety. Most of the machines are designed to assist you through the process of lifting and have safety devices to protect you from harm. Unlike free weights—or handheld weights for that matter—weight-lifting machines regulate pressure, force, and balance. The machine typically has only one way to use it, whereas with handheld weights you have a myriad of options. But when you use a machine, you don't need a spotter helping you.

NOTE: A spotter is always a good idea even if it isn't necessary. Besides helping you be safe, a workout partner can push you harder than you would by yourself.

Weigh out (pun intended) the pros and cons and determine which is best for you. Often it is a combination of all that works best.

Body Basics

No matter what type of resistance program you select, you need to ensure that you are eating enough protein and drinking plenty of water (more nutrition information is available in chapter nine.) Our muscles consist of 70 percent water and 30 percent protein, so you can see how important it is to have these two elements in your diet.[3] Eliminate these, and you are damaging your muscles.

Now let's talk about the specific muscles in your body for a moment. I don't want to bog you down with every single one, because that would take too many pages of text. I do, however, want to point out the major muscle groups that you should be concentrating on during your workout. Focus on these, and you will get a complete body workout:

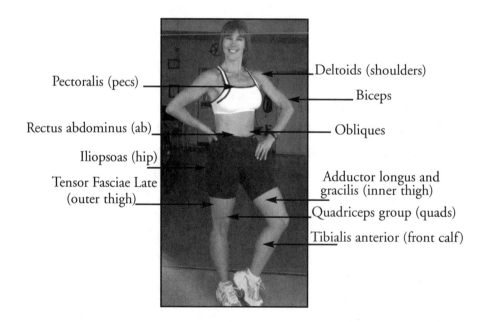

Pectoralis (pecs)

Rectus abdominus (ab)

Iliopsoas (hip)

Tensor Fasciae Late (outer thigh)

Deltoids (shoulders)

Biceps

Obliques

Adductor longus and gracilis (inner thigh)

Quadriceps group (quads)

Tibialis anterior (front calf)

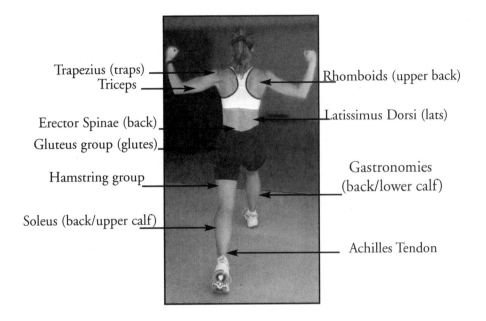

Trapezius (traps)
Triceps
Erector Spinae (back)
Gluteus group (glutes)
Hamstring group
Soleus (back/upper calf)

Rhomboids (upper back)
Latissimus Dorsi (lats)
Gastronomies (back/lower calf)
Achilles Tendon

Always exercise opposing muscles

Notice that I've pointed out the muscles of the back of the body, not just the front. Sometimes we concentrate on the front of the body because we see it. It is very important to include the muscles in the backside of the body, which are the *opposing* muscles. Our bodies are divided into front and back sections (anterior and posterior). For every muscle on the front of your body, you have an opposing or posterior muscle. If you work your arm (bicep) muscle, then you must remember to also exercise the back of your arm (triceps).

People often forget this basic principle and injure themselves. For example, a tennis player who focuses more on building up his quads and forgets to work his hamstrings is more likely to pull a hamstring when he reaches to get a ball. Why? His quads are overpowering his hamstrings and pulling on them. Because his hamstrings are weaker than his quads, they cannot sustain the tension and they pull. And it hurts, too!

In order to prevent injury and simply balance your body, be sure to work the following muscles equally:

Chart 5.1—Upper and Lower Body Opposing Muscles

Primary Muscles (Anterior)	Opposing Muscles (Posterior)
UPPER BODY	
Pecs	Traps/Rhomboids
Biceps	Triceps
Abs	Erector spinae (back)
Obliques	Lats
LOWER BODY	
Hips	Glutes
Quads	Hamstrings
Tibialis anterior (front calf)	Gastrocnemius/soleus (back calf)

Inner/outer thigh

A great way to work both your inner and outer thigh muscles at the same time is to do side leg lifts on the floor.

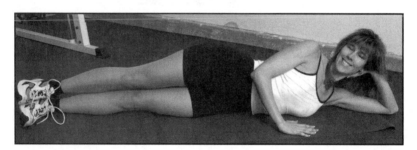

Lie down on your side, and stack both legs on top of each other. Align your body so that you are in a straight line. (Shoulder, hip, and ankle should be in alignment.) Use a hand in front of your body on the floor if you need additional stability. With your feet facing forward, begin to slowly lift your top leg.

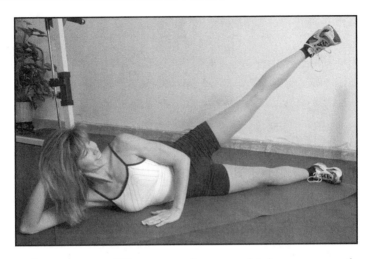

Breathe out as you lift your top leg up as high as you can, keeping the bottom leg on the floor at all times. Concentrate on keeping the movements controlled. You will feel this in your outer thigh and hip area. Breathe in as you slowly lower your leg back to the starting position, without plopping it down. Count to ten (that is, do ten reps), or however many you want to do, which is one set.

Stay where you are, but bend the top leg and swing it around to the front of your body and grab your ankle for support. You will now keep that leg in position and move the bottom leg up.

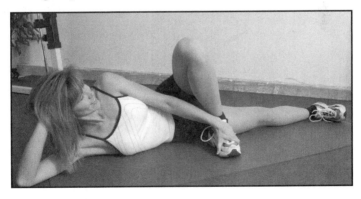

This will really work your inner thigh muscle. The inner thigh is the opposing muscle for the outer thigh. This exercise allows you to alternate between the two easily.

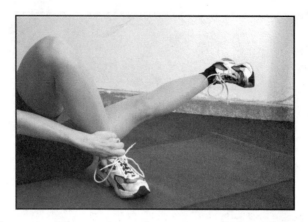

Exhale as you lift your lower leg up toward the ceiling, again raising it as high as you can. Do not be discouraged if it is not very high off the ground. These muscles are not worked that often and may be weak. If, however, you find it easy to lift, add the weight of your other leg as additional resistance. Maintain that straight alignment with your feet facing forward.

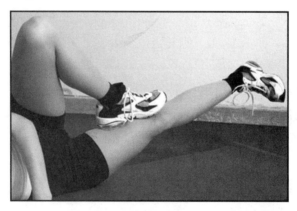

NOTE: Again, these are a great option for any age and ability level. You can add ankle weights to increase the resistance.

Don't overuse

CAUTION: Be careful not to fall into a dull routine in your weight lifting. Changing it up not only keeps it fun and creative (thus preventing boredom, which is the number one reason people stop exercising[4]), but it also prevents injury. If you continually perform the same exercise week after week, you are subjecting yourself to the possibility of repetitive damage. You want to work all the muscles out each week, but do it in a different manner. Try new ways and new toys! They all work different core muscles as well. We have so many fun exercise devices now that you can really have a "ball." OK, I'll stop with the puns.

One way to change up your workout is to adapt the same exercise. Push-ups, for example, can be done in three levels. Level one is done on all fours (hands and knees), and you concentrate on lowering just the upper body toward the floor.

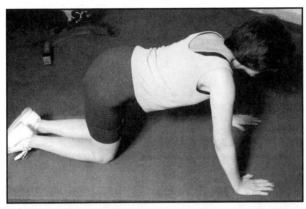

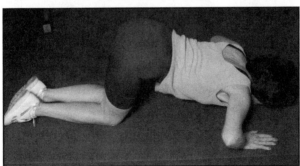

Level two is done with your knees back with a greater degree of reach, and you lower more of your body down toward the floor.

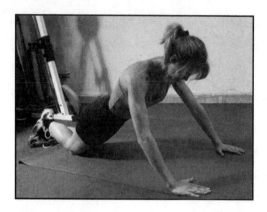

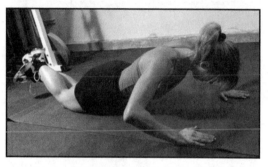

Level three is the traditional, full-body push-up that you are most familiar with.

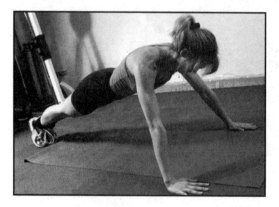

Depending upon the day and how strong your core muscles are, choose the level that works best for you.

Let's get to the core

Speaking of core muscles, I can't show you a picture of them unless we had a technical drawing, but even then, they are so deep with our body that they are difficult to see. But just because we can't see them doesn't mean they aren't vital to our health. These puppies help us stand, sit, balance, and so on. Our abs and erector spinae (back) are two of the largest and most important core muscles we have, so these are the core muscles we will focus on in this book.

For years, these muscles were forgotten. Many clients who were athletes in their youth are astounded by the core muscle workouts I give them and wish they had known about them twenty years ago. It is your core muscles that assist *all* of your other muscles. If they are strong, you will be even better at whatever you are doing. If, however, they are weak, then you will see slower gains. Core muscles are like the foundation of a house. When it is solid, the house stands. But if the foundation is cracked or compromised, the entire house is ruined. We all must include these core muscles in our workouts for total health.

You are probably wondering how to find out if you have weak core muscles. Research indicates that 80 percent of Americans suffer from back pain, which is a direct result of weak core muscles.[5] To determine how strong your core is, take this simple test.

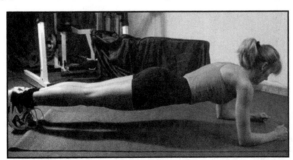

Get down on the floor, and lie facedown. Put your weight on your elbows and your toes, keeping a completely straight line from your toes to your head. How long can you hold this? If it is literally just seconds, then you have weak core muscles. If you can hold it for a minute or longer, then your core muscles are in decent shape. The longer you can sustain the position, the better. This is also a great core stretch to practice on a regular basis. See if you can extend the amount of time you stay up in position.

NOTE: If you have had back problems or have joint pain, I suggest you try one of the other core strengthening techniques instead.

Here are some other examples of ways you can build your core strength, which will improve your overall health and performance.

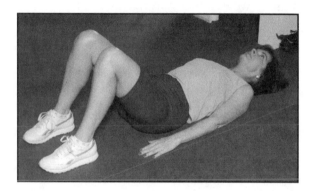

This core muscle exercise is not only working your abs and erector spinae, but it is ALSO strengthening your glutes and legs. Start off by lying on your back with your arms to your side. Your knees are bent with your feet flat on the floor. Concentrate on pushing your abs through to the floor, through your back. Your back should be pressed against the floor and your abs flat and firm. The key to this exercise is to proceed slowly with control.

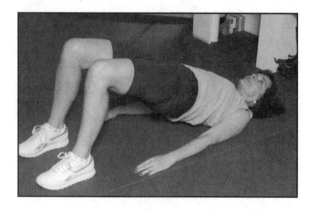

Begin lifting your tailbone up off the ground and continue to lift one vertebra at a time. Considering we have twenty-six vertebrae, this should take you at least thirty seconds. Once your shoulder blades are lifted off the ground, hold this "tabletop" position for a count of ten. Then slowly lower your body down in reverse, one vertebra at a time. You should feel your core muscles working hard to stabilize you.

Your body will want to plop down on the ground. Don't let it! Resist. Breathe slowly, and really concentrate. Repeat this up to eight times for a superb core-strengthening exercise.

Superman

Another great back-strengthening exercise from the floor is what I call the Superman. Lie on your stomach with your arms straight out as if you're flying and your legs straight out behind you. Keep your head looking down at the floor.

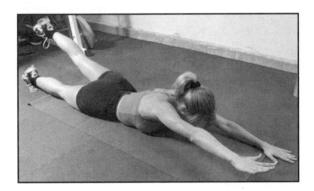

Lift your right arm and left leg at the same time, then lower. Then lift your left arm and right leg, and lower. That is one rep. Keep alternating, and do ten reps.

You can also work on posture while working your back muscle by sitting on the floor with your legs out in front of you.

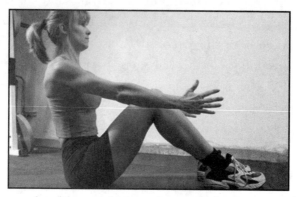

Lean your shoulders and chest forward, forcing your back to be straight and upright. Hold your arms out in front of you, and hold that for a count of twenty or thirty seconds.

Leanback

An exercise not only excellent for building stronger core muscles, but also for stretching your shoulders and hamstrings is what I call the lean-back. Start off sitting on the floor with your legs out in front of you, pressed against the floor. Stack up your spine nice and straight, and begin to lean back, one vertebra at a time. As you lean back, maintain control and do not allow gravity to pull you down quickly. Once you are lying flat on your back, reach your arms up over your head to stretch your shoulders out. Take in a couple of breaths.

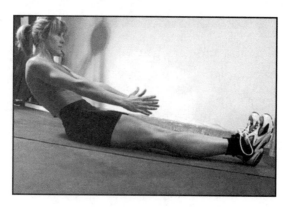

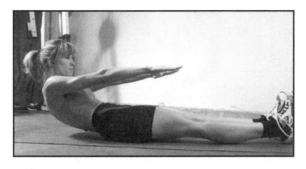

Now lift your head and look at your toes. Begin to bring your torso up, one vertebra at a time, reaching your arms forward. Stack your spine back up, and reach for your toes; touch them if possible. Pause here for a moment, and stretch out your hamstrings by grabbing on to your toes, but do not pull on them. Stack your spine back up, and repeat this process several times.

Ways you can adapt this exercise to meet your needs: (1) Bend your knees instead of keeping them straight. (2) Have a workout buddy hold your feet to give you a little stability.

Another option

An option that is a bit easier on the back is the extended toe reach. Lying on your back, extend your legs up to a ninety-degree angle. Reach your right hand toward your left toe without moving your legs and then your left hand to your right toe. Keep alternating.

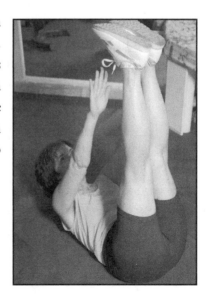

After you have counted to ten (remember, one of each side equals one rep), spread your legs wide, keeping them as straight as possible without locking your knees. Reach your arms to the outside of your legs (left arm to left side and right arm to the right side). Let your arms pulse (bounce gently), and remember to breathe slowly. Count to ten.

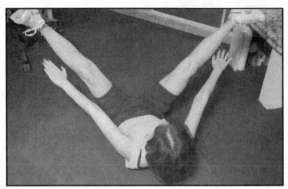

Building core strength should be woven into your fitness program. Most seasoned veteran classes are incorporating yoga, Pilates, or PiYo, which is a combination of the two. Give it a try; I know you will be pleased with the results. One student of mine had severe back pain. After weeks of incorporating the tabletop exercise one vertebra at a time, he had more back movement and less pain.

Specific weight-training goals

Each person reading this book will have different goals. I would like to outline for you, though, some basics to help get you started. Your age, lifestyle, and current health will influence your goals.

Chart 5.2—Personalize Your Weight-Training Goals

AGE	OBJECTIVE	REPS/SETS	WEIGHTS USED	FREQUENCY
All	Maintenance program	15 reps/2 sets	Lighter weights	2–3/week
All	Healthy muscles and bones	10 reps/2 sets	Lighter weights	2–3/week
40–60	Tone and define muscles	10 reps/3 sets	Medium weights	2–3/week
40–60	Reduce body fat	12 reps/3 sets	Medium weights	2–3/week
40–60	Increase muscle mass	8 reps/3 sets	Heavy weights	3–4/week
55 and older	Reduce joint pain/arthritis	8–10 reps/2 sets	Light weights or bands	3–4/week
70 and older	Mobility/ functionality	8 reps/2 sets	Bands	3–4/week

Be sure to look at the chapter for your specific age group for additional program ideas and pictures!

DON'T FORGET TO STRETCH

Most seasoned veterans have learned the importance of stretching. Stretching after you have worked your muscles hard allows them to perform again. Without stretching, you are limiting their potential and setting yourself up for injury. Tight muscles may pull on the bone the wrong way, thus causing you to trip or fall. Don't forget to weave this into any fitness program you do, as it is paramount to our overall health and well-being.

HOW OFTEN SHOULD I STRETCH?

You should stretch every time you exercise. Warm yourself up before you exercise, and then stretch yourself out when you are done.

When your muscles are engaged in activity, they require more blood. The body sends this blood to them in their time of need. However, when you cease activity, the muscles no longer need extra blood. In order to return this blood to where it started, you must stretch the muscles out and release it. If you don't, it can pool up in that muscle and, in severe cases, cause blood clots.[6] It isn't worth the risk. Stretch!

Most seasoned veteran classes have a good amount of stretching in them, but I encourage you to stretch additionally throughout the week.

You should stretch every time you exercise.

Trust me; once you begin stretching you'll get hooked! One gal from my class had horrible hip pain for years and years. She tried everything and visited many doctors. After attending my class three times a week for six months and stretching her hip and leg, her pain disappeared!

What Kind of Stretching Should I Do?

All stretching is not created equal. There are three types of stretching: ballistic, rhythmic limbering, and static.[7]

Ballistic is the type of stretch where you bounce through it—pulse, if you will. Studies have shown that this type of stretch is not safe for the general public, especially older populations.[8] It can cause more harm than good, so I discourage you from doing it.

Instead, try rhythmic limbering stretching. This is what most aerobic classes include in their warm-up stage. Rhythmic limbering warms up the exact muscles you expect to utilize in a workout. You are performing the actual movements you'll use later, but at a lesser degree.

For example, if you are a golfer or tennis player who used rhythmic limbering, you wouldn't hold your stretches before playing.

Rather, you would imitate your swing without the club or racquet. This is preparing the appropriate muscles for the game ahead. When you add the club or racquet and intensity of the game, then it gets worked out. It's at the conclusion of your game when you would hold stretches for your arms, shoulders, and legs.

This method of stretching that holds the stretch is called a static stretch. Hold it for a few seconds, breathing through. If you were stretching your quad after playing tennis, for instance, you would bring your heel back toward your glute with your knee pointing straight down. Keep your legs aligned, and hold it for a few seconds, breathing slowly.

Resistance training can make your muscles tight. It's the natural process of contracting. You can see it if you pay attention. After lifting weights, your muscles look bigger and stronger. They are firm. If you don't stretch them out, then over time they may stay hard. This will cause them to shorten, and you will lose flexibility. This can cause problems and injuries down the road. Think of stretching as preventative maintenance. We get our cars serviced to avoid trouble, and stretching and cooling your body down after working out will do the same.

How Long Do I Need To Stretch?

How long you stretch will be determined by what activity you performed. See below for some suggestions:

- Aerobics/seasoned veterans' classes—Your warm-up should include both limbering and static stretches for approximately five to ten minutes, especially if you are to perform high-power moves. Your cool down (usually five to eight minutes) should start off with limbering moves until the heart rate declines slightly, then static stretch the lower and upper body as well as the back.

- Tennis/golf/sports—Warm up with static stretches of the quad, hamstring, and inner/outer thigh muscles.

Use rhythmic limbering movements for the upper body (swinging the arms and rotating the shoulder) just for two to three minutes. Cool down longer at the end with static stretches for lower and upper body, approximately five minutes.

NOTE: If you can include additional days of just stretching, you will see pain disappear due to greater flexibility. Some terrific ways to incorporate this into your routine is by using Pilates and yoga. Just remember to breathe through. Take deep breaths, and allow the muscle to release and relax.

Stretching should feel warm, but it should not hurt. If your muscle starts to shake on you, don't worry. It means you are stretching deep and that muscle was very tight. You are doing the right thing! But like everything else, if you experience pain, STOP immediately.

STRETCH YOURSELF

I know many people are not used to stretching or have not taken the time in the past, but here are some great ones for you:

Arm stretch series

For this series sit Indian style if you can, or in any position that is comfortable for you.

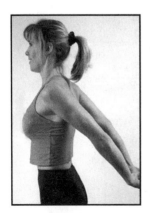

Standing (or sitting) up nice and tall, move your arms behind you and grab your hands together. Your arms should be just about straight, but do not lock your elbows. Raise your arms up as high as you can go while keeping your head looking forward. This stretches out your shoulders and pecs.

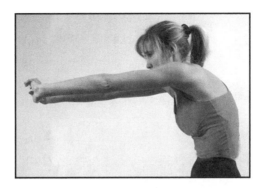

Now, curve your spine and bring your arms forward, looking down. Press your wrists out away from your body. This will stretch your lats, rhomboids, and upper back. Remember to breathe in and out as you hold this stretch for at least twenty seconds.

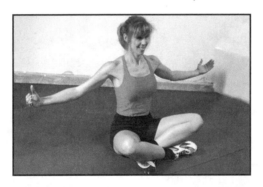

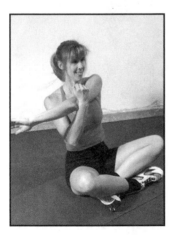

Sit up nice and tall again. Spread your arms wide. Bring your left arm across the front to the other side. With your left thumb facing the floor, bring your right arm over and push your left elbow to extend the stretch. Hold it here, and breathe in and out for twenty seconds. This will stretch out your biceps and shoulders. Switch arms, and reverse the stretch. Hold again for twenty seconds, breathing deeply all the while.

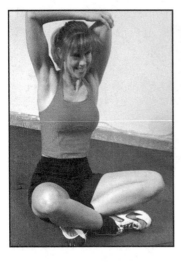

The last arm stretch in this series will get your triceps and shoulders/deltoids. Sitting nice and tall again, bring one arm back over your shoulder as if giving yourself a pat on the back. Your other hand will push on your elbow, helping that arm go down your back. Keep your head looking forward to reduce strain on the neck. Breathe in and out, and hold the stretch for twenty seconds. Switch arms, and you are done with your upper body.

Leg stretch series

Now on to your legs. I love this series. It's the one that has helped my clients and class members the most. You will need a stretchy band, jump rope, or Pilates ring.

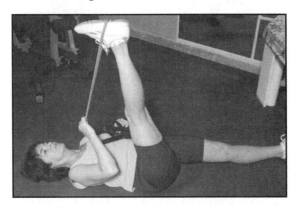

Start off by lying on your back on the floor. Both legs will be straight out. Step one heel into the band, holding it with both hands. Bring the leg in the band up, and keep the other leg flat on the floor. Bring the leg up as far as you can, keeping it straight but without locking the knee. Your head should remain on the floor. Relax, and let the warmth of this stretch settle in to your quads and hamstrings. Keep breathing, and hold the stretch for thirty seconds.

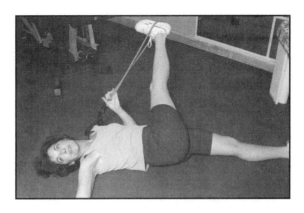

Now allow the leg that is up to cross over toward the opposite side of your body. Depending upon your flexibility, you may be able to get close to the ground, but don't touch it. Keep your shoulders square on the floor. This is an awesome stretch for your hips and lower back. Breathe in and out, and hold this for thirty seconds. Switch legs and repeat. Not only does this help your muscles release and prepare for the next workout, but it also helps prevent muscle soreness.

Stress-reduction/tension-headache-reducing stretch

The next stretch may sound silly and actually look funny, but it sure beats getting a migraine or tension headache.

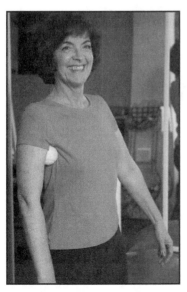

You will need two tennis balls. I prefer to wear a t-shirt rather than a sleeveless top for this one, but either will work. Place a tennis ball under each armpit. Square your shoulders, and stand up straight. By holding those balls in place and preventing them from moving, you are perfectly aligned. This is good posture! Most of us are not used to it, so you may feel the back muscles working a bit. Walk around for five to ten minutes like this, and feel the tension release from your upper back and neck. This elongates those muscles and helps them relax. Keep your head up and forward.

If you spend a lot of time in front of a computer, I highly recommend you do this as often as possible.

SEEING IS BELIEVING!

Whew! That was an awful lot of information at once, wasn't it? The good news is that you can reference this chapter any time! In fact, I encourage you to reread this after you have spent time with your specific stage of life chapter.

Don't be discouraged, either. This may all be overwhelming right now because it is new to you, but the more you do it, the more comfortable you will become. Practice makes perfect! The chapter for your specific age bracket will have even more photos to illustrate exercise options for *you*. I know visuals help, and seeing is believing! So what are we waiting for? Let's move on!

FIT

Section Three

Fitness Is for You!

50

Chapter Six

Physical Fitness for Forty- to Fifty-Five-Year-Olds

Do you remember when "backing up" was something you did with your car in a parking lot? Do you recall the days when a "bug" was the reason you called in sick? How about a time when a "chip" was yummy to eat? If you think "networking" is something you do with a group of people at a business function, you might be "pre-personal computer." You might even be pre-electric typewriter! I learned to type on a manual typewriter that required pressing down really hard on every key, and I remember the day when IBM introduced their IBM Selectric typewriter. Wow, what a machine! It sure beat correction liquid and tape.

Just as technology has changed around us, so our bodies are also starting to show signs of changing times. Now if only we didn't have to continue getting pimples when the wrinkles come—that doesn't seem fair to me at all!

In section two we covered some basics about the aging process and got an introduction into cardiovascular exercise and resistance training. Section three is the heart of *Fit Over 50*. Here we will discuss optimum fitness plans for three age brackets in the seasoned veterans category: forty to fifty-five (this chapter), fifty-six to sixty-five (chapter seven), and sixty-six-plus (chapter eight).

Even though it is never too late to begin exercising, the younger a person starts, the more strength that can be gained. Congratulations on starting today. I'm proud of you. The more you do now, the more you will be able to do later, which can improve not only your quantity but also your quality of living.

Stages of Life

At this stage of life (forty to fifty-five years old), you may find yourself doing a variety of activities simply because you enjoy them. Perhaps your children are older, and you are able to spend more time on your own interests: sailing, golf, tennis, traveling, and so on. If you started your family later in life, you may still have children at home. If this is the case, you might be participating in activities with them such as dirt bike riding, hiking, biking, camping, and the like. Children grow up so quickly—take advantage of every moment. Maybe you are fortunate enough to be retired already. Good for you! The world is your oyster.

No matter what your situation, these years are very important for your long-term health. Make the time to care for yourself regardless of your situation.

This chapter is dedicated to you: forty- to fifty-five-year-olds. Together, we will customize an exercise program that will fit into your busy life without boring you.

These years are paramount for building strength, for if you do not do it now, you may not have the opportunity later. The younger the body is, the better it responds to muscle building, but of course any age can benefit from strength training. And the younger you are, the harder you can push your body in cardiovascular exercise as well.

Use your strength to your advantage, and increase your performance so that you have more to work with later in life. Schedule your exercise time (both cardio and resistance training) on your calendar just as you would any other appointment.

Get Your Cardiovascular Exercise In

Here are some cardio programs that are likely to be a good match for your stage of life. The intensity column refers back to the Workout Intensity Chart on page 54. Find what works for you and your lifestyle.

Chart 6.1—Cardio Programs for Forty- to Fifty-Five-Year-Olds

Exercise	Frequency	Intensity
Running—indoor or on treadmill	3–5 times a week	Level 8–8$\frac{1}{2}$ (Visit 9 briefly, but you'll want to keep most of the run at level 8.)
Jogging outside	3–5 times a week	Level 8–8$\frac{1}{2}$ (Visit 9, but try to keep the majority of your jog at an 8.)
Indoor cycling	3 times a week	Level 8–8$\frac{1}{2}$ (Visit 9, but try to keep the majority of your workout at an 8.)
Outdoor cycling	3–5 times a week	Level 8–8$\frac{1}{2}$ (Visit 9, but try to keep the majority of your ride at level 8.)
Swimming	3–5 times a week	Level 8–8$\frac{1}{2}$ (Visit 9, but try to keep the majority of your swim at an 8.)
Seasoned veterans class	3 times a week	Level 8–8$\frac{1}{2}$ (Visit 9, but you will most likely stay at level 8.)
Circuit class	3 times a week	Level 8–8$\frac{1}{2}$ (Visit 9, but keep your workload mostly at 8 and 8$\frac{1}{2}$.)
Tennis	3–5 times a week	Level 8–8$\frac{1}{2}$
Jumping rope	3–5 times a week	Level 8–8$\frac{1}{2}$ (You will easily get to 9 if you pick up the pace at which you jump—just be sure to stay at 8 most of the time.)
Elliptical machine	3–5 times a week	Level 8–8$\frac{1}{2}$ (Visit 9 for a bit, but keep the rest of your time at 8.)

Time	Tips for Your Stage
20 minutes at level 8 30 minutes total	If you are already a runner, keep on keeping on! To protect your joints, add a treadmill run every once in a while (or sand). Monitor your pace and breathing for a great workout.
20 minutes at level 8 30 minutes total	No need to "run" if you are not used to it. A steady jog will do the trick, but make sure to incorporate hills to get that intensity up.
1 hour	Most classes are one hour in length. Try a variety of instructors and types: climbs, hills, all-terrain, and endurance. NOTE: Cycle shorts or gel seats help with comfort.
At least 30 minutes	If you are a cyclist, you love being outside. But this is a great way to exercise even for the novice cyclist. Map out routes with some hills to challenge you. Just remember that you have to ride back!
20–30 minutes	Dive in, swim your laps, and get out. It's a fast, effective workout as it really builds your upper body strength without impact.
1 hour	These classes are designed to be low impact. If you require a harder workload, raise your arms, take wider steps, and add some impact. Besides being a great workout, these classes are typically fun and provide a social outlet.
1 hour	These classes, like the seasoned veterans class, combine cardio with sculpting. They are a great way to get both cardio and resistance training in. This is individualized because you pick your own weight level.
At least 30 minutes	Most matches are $1\frac{1}{2}$–2 hours in length. Singles will give you a better workout, but doubles can be more fun. Whichever you prefer, this is an excellent way to get outside and get in shape.
8–15 minutes	Eight minutes is an eternity with a jump rope, and it may take you a lot of practice to build up to it. This is an intensive workout that maximizes time. Switch up how you jump or add music to make it more enjoyable. This is a perfect indoor option for bad weather days.
20 minutes at level 8; 30 minutes total	Another indoor option that is easy on the joints. Just make sure to keep the intensity up. You should be moving fast enough to prevent reading or talking.

Exercise	Frequency	Intensity
Sports teams	1–3 times a week	Level 8–$8^1/_2$ (Some sports make it hard to maintain this level long enough for health benefit.)
Hiking, canoeing, etc.	1–3 times a week	Level 8–$8^1/_2$ (Visit 9 when possible.)
Step and other aerobic classes	3–5 times a week	Level 8–$8^1/_2$ (Visit 9, but spend the majority of the class at 8.)

You may have something else you like to do, and that's great. These are just suggestions that will help you get enough cardiovascular exercise in—and at the right intensity—so that you experience a health benefit.

I encourage you to set a schedule that you can count on. In fact, work around your workout schedule if you can. Many of my seasoned veteran participants plan on their class every Monday, Wednesday, and Friday. Appointments are arranged around their classes. Only emergencies and rare situations take them away. Sound too serious? Your health *is* a serious issue. Treat it with care and respect. Do not wait until you lose it to appreciate how important it is.

Time	Tips for Your Stage
At least 30 minutes	These are fun activities, but they don't always provide an intense enough workout, so don't rely solely on them. Variety is the key.
At least 30 minutes	Outdoor activities are a superb way to enjoy your family and get exercise. Most schedules don't permit enough of these to keep up with cardio requirements, so weave in other options. But don't forget them!
1 hour	A variety of classes exists for awesome cardio work. Beware of advanced classes that torque knees and overuse the back, such as kickboxing. If you participate, use caution and adapt the moves as necessary.

Cardio program log

Below is a chart you can use to schedule and track your cardiovascular workouts. I encourage you to use it as an accountability partner or success record. Regardless of whether you find it easy or challenging to get plenty of activity each week, this program log helps you plan your exercise and protect it.

On the log, *cardio mode* refers to the type of exercise you choose to engage in from the cardio program chart (running, swimming, jumping rope, and the like). Make copies of this form, and use it when you are working out. Keep it in your day planner or on your refrigerator. Find what works for you, and *do it!*

Chart 6.2—Cardio Program Log

DAY/DATE	MODE	TIME	INTENSITY	NOTES
Monday				
Tuesday				
Wednesday				
Thursday				
Friday				
Saturday				
Sunday				
Monday				
Tuesday				
Wednesday				
Thursday				
Friday				
Saturday				
Sunday				
Monday				
Tuesday				
Wednesday				
Thursday				
Friday				
Saturday				
Sunday				
Monday				
Tuesday				
Wednesday				
Thursday				
Friday				
Saturday				
Sunday				

Monday				
Tuesday				
Wednesday				
Thursday				
Friday				
Saturday				
Sunday				
Monday				
Tuesday				
Wednesday				
Thursday				
Friday				
Saturday				
Sunday				
Monday				
Tuesday				
Wednesday				
Thursday				
Friday				
Saturday				
Sunday				

Adapt as necessary

No matter what type of exercise you choose, remember to work at your own level and adapt accordingly. Most fitness classes will offer several levels of intensity, allowing you to pick the workout that is right for you. Here are some ways for you to adapt the intensity level of the exercises I have recommended for your cardio workout:

Chart 6.3—Customize Your Intensity Level (Ages Forty to Forty-Five)

Exercise	Low Intensity (Levels 1–4)	Medium Intensity (Levels 5–7)
Running—indoor or on treadmill	Flat, short course (1–3 miles)	Longer course or rolling hills/increase grade on treadmill (3–5 miles)
Jogging outside	Flat, short course (1–3 miles)	Longer course or rolling hills (3–5 miles)
Indoor cycling	Endurance class or beginner (remain seated)	Climbing/strength class or intermediate
Outdoor cycling	Flat, short course (8–10 miles)	Longer course with rolling hills (10–15 miles)
Swimming	Indoor pool laps	Lake swim
Seasoned veterans class	Arms down, legs close together, side steps, no impact	Arms up, legs further apart, higher lifts
Circuit class	Light weights, no impact (see above)	Medium weights, legs farther apart (see above)
Tennis	Mixed doubles	Doubles
Jumping rope	One leg at a time, soft kick or swing forward	Both legs together as you jump
Elliptical machine	Slow cadence without arms	Medium cadence with arms
Sports teams	Family team or church league	Coed recreational team
Hiking, canoeing, etc.	Easy, flat, calm trails or routes	All terrain trails or routes
Step and other aerobic classes	No risers, arms to side, legs close together, side steps, grapevine, no kicks	1 riser, arms up, legs farther apart, low kicks, side lift, grapevine with curl

High Intensity (Levels 8–10)	Notes
Longer course or hills/ increase grade on treadmill (5–8 miles)	You can increase speed without changing the distance. For example, run a 10-minute mile instead of a 12-minute mile.
Longer course or hills (5–8 miles)	If you increase your speed on any level, you increase the intensity. Before you turn your jog into a run, make sure you have supportive shoes.
All-terrain class or difficult	All are one hour in length.
Longer course with hills (15–50 miles)	You can change this up even more by racing, which takes the intensity up.
Ocean swim	Make sure you have the right gear for cold-water swimming.
Arms up, legs farther apart; add impact (full jumping jacks)	Don't push too hard too fast. The good news is that you can take it down at any time you need to. Every day is different. Don't expect to perform at the same level all the time.
Heavier weights, add impact (see above)	The more workload you put on your muscles, the greater the intensity.
Singles	Singles provides the greatest workout, although doubles can be pretty competitive.
Both legs together, side-to-side jumping, or power jumping (swing the rope twice for every jump)	This is an intensive workout in either case. Want to take it even lower? Forgo the rope and imitate the action. It's still a good workout.
Fast cadence with arms	The quicker you go, the better the workout. See what you can do. Challenge yourself a little bit each time. Step by step.
Competitive league	Any sport you like has a variety of levels to play. Pick the one that fits you and is fun!
Difficult/advanced trails and routes	Do your homework before embarking on outdoor activities. Heed the ratings systems, and come prepared.
2 risers or more, arms up, legs further apart, kicks, knees up, grapevine with jump and curl	The instructor should demonstrate different levels for you. At any time, you can change levels. Be safe.

Here is an example of Tim adapting how high he brings up his knee and arms in a cardio class. One is lower intensity than the other, but they are both good options.

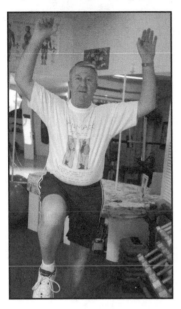
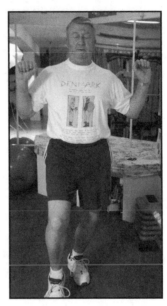

WEIGHT LIFTING

Exercise must also include resistance training, as I have explained earlier. And because these are your strength-building years, take advantage of your ability to push harder. Later in life you may need to reduce your weights, but right now I encourage you to increase them. Remember: the stronger your muscles, the healthier your bones. Eventually, our bones will start to lose mass. The bigger they are to begin with, the better off you will be.

Which weight is right for you?

If you have been lifting weights already, you should have a good idea of which weight works for you. I challenge you, though, to make sure you are not "settling." We often *can* lift more than we *do* lift. It may take a little more work, but that's the idea!

If you've never lifted before, start off easy. Find a weight that is difficult enough to push you but not too heavy to hurt you. Once you get your starting point, you will have established your benchmark. From there, you will either continue on with the same weight or increase it as you become stronger. Spend time evaluating each muscle and trying a variety of weights.

For example, a woman may start off with only five-pound hand weights for her bicep curl. She should be able to increase this to eight pounds and eventually ten pounds. She may stay at the ten or press harder for twelve or fifteen pounds. Take the two weights together (one in each hand, remember), and you have a pretty heavy load. Men are traditionally stronger because they have more testosterone and more muscle fibers. They should be able to lift eight to ten to start and build from there. Men can find themselves upwards of thirty to fifty pounds per hand if they work at it.

Partner up

When at all possible, lift with a buddy. Partners are important for exercises that could harm you. For example, people have been crushed under a bar when performing a bench press alone. Be safe, or you could find yourself in trouble. Don't feel bad if you start off with lower weights. Remember, small steps! Any resistance training is better than none. If your muscles have not been worked before, they will be weak. This is a fact. But the exciting news is that your body will respond quickly. Before you know it you will be getting stronger and healthier.

Caution

During any exercise, whether cardiovascular or weight lifting, if you experience pain, stop! Your body is telling you something. It is better to listen up front to your body's whisper than experience it screaming at you later. A little prevention will help you stay at it longer. Pain is often an indicator of too much, too soon.

If you feel pain when doing cardio exercise (muscle pain, not breathing complications), simply reduce your impact, lower your arms, or walk in place. With weight lifting, lower the amount of weight until you eventually build yourself up to a heavier weight. If at any time you experience symptoms remotely close to a heart attack, seek medical attention immediately.

This does not mean you should never feel anything uncomfortable. If you are embarking on a new fitness program, you *will* feel it. You will experience some soreness and muscle fatigue. This is part of the process. If you follow the guidelines in this book, however, such discomfort should be minimal. But nonetheless, it is par for the course when starting a new workout routine.

I mentioned earlier that I highly suggest you seek the counsel of a physician before you start your new program. I can't emphasize this enough, especially if you are overweight or have been living a sedentary lifestyle. If you have a family history of heart disease or other restrictive ailments, you definitely need to get a checkup and overall physical before you begin. Better to be safe than sorry!

Weight-lifting strength log

Just like your cardio exercise, I suggest you log your resistance training. Besides, this chart ensures that you don't forget a muscle. I spend every day training people, and I still use this log.

Chart 6.4—Weight-Lifting Strength Log
(Forty- to Fifty-Five-Year-Olds)

Muscle	Mode	Seat/ Settings	Weight/ Reps #1	Weight/ Reps #2	Weight/ Reps #3	Stretch?
Quads						
Hamstrings						
Glutes						
Calves						
Inner thigh						
Outer thigh						
Forearms, hands						
Biceps						
Triceps						
Shoulders						
Deltoids						
Pecs						
Lats/ rhomboids						
Erector spinae						
Abs						
Obliques						

WEIGHT-LIFTING EXERCISES FOR SPECIFIC MUSCLE GROUPS

I was quite pleased with a compliment a client gave me the other day. He said, "Gee, Lorraine, I've been coming to see you for three months now, and we haven't done the same exercise twice!" First of all, I personally like variety, and I knew my client would appreciate it as well. Second, changing up our exercises helps prevent overuse and injury. The following pages will show you a variety of exercises that you can incorporate into your personal workout. Here's to working those muscles to good health!

The following exercises use a combination of floor work, free weights, and exercise machines. Each one works a major muscle.

Quads

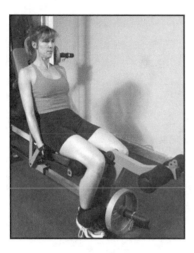

The leg extension is a pretty standard movement.

You start seated with your back supported. Hold on to the handrails or bottom of your seat for stability. Your feet go under the bar (toes up), and you lift the bar up with your legs. Breathe out as you lift it up to the point where your legs are almost straight, but don't lock your knees.

You should feel this on the top of your leg. Your knees will be worked, but you should not experience sharp pain. If you do, immediately stop. Check your seat settings to ensure that you are not too far forward. And make sure you haven't tried to lift too much weight too soon.

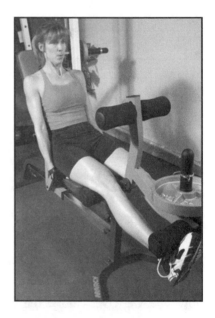

Another great option that does not require any equipment is what I call "sitting against the wall," because that is exactly what you do. Press your back and bottom against the wall, and sink down until you make a 90-degree angle. Hold the position, but keep breathing. I like to squeeze a stress ball or something while I do this to take my mind off the workload on the top of the legs. Do you feel it? Oh, yeah, this is a good one. Try to go fifteen seconds, twenty seconds, and then thirty seconds. This is a position we'll use for the rest of our lives, so it is a good one to weave in.

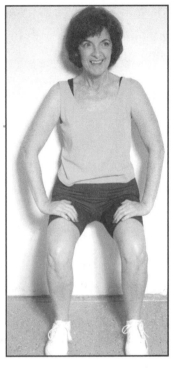

NOTE: Another great leg workout is lunges. Lunges work all three leg muscle groups (quads, hamstrings, and glutes) and can vary in their level of difficulty. See chapter seven for pictures—and remember to watch your form.

Hamstrings

The hamstrings are the muscles at the back of your leg. To work this group of muscles, you curl your legs instead of extending them.

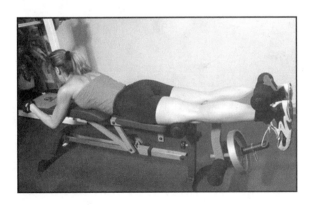

Start off by lying on your stomach with your hips pressed into the machine. Put your heels behind the bar and curl your them into your glute, breathing out. Hold on to the bench or machine, and keep your hips pressed against it. If you find your rear lifting up and your hips moving, you probably have too much weight. Typically, we are weaker on the backside of our body since it does not get everyday use. So don't worry if it is less than what you can lift with your quads. That's normal.

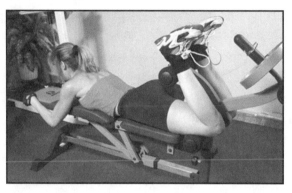

Another way to work this muscle group and your calves at the same time is to curl in on an exercise ball.

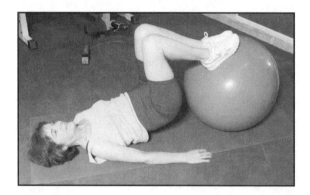

You will need an exercise ball and a floor mat. Lying down on your back, face up, put your heels on the ball. Lift your bottom up off the ground to create a tabletop.

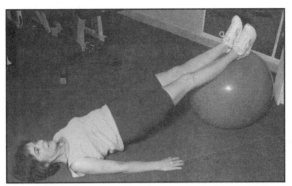

By the way, this is an excellent way to work your core muscles, too. Hold that tabletop, and never let your bottom touch the ground. Now, bring your heels toward your glutes, keeping the toes pointing up to the ceiling. Breathe out as you curl in, and breathe in as you extend your legs. You'll want to take a rest break between sets.

Glutes

Although sitting on our rears doesn't do us any good, the motion of sitting down is an excellent workout for one of your largest muscle groups: your glutes.

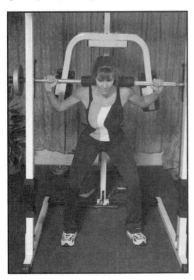

The movement in this exercise is called a squat, and it is just like sitting down. You have your legs apart, feet forward, and you reach behind you with your bottom. Think of it as aiming for the seat cushion but holding yourself above the chair. Your heels should be flat on the floor. If you lift your heels, you'll put too much strain on your knees. This movement can be done with a machine, as shown, or with hand weights for additional resistance. Still too much? You can put all weights down and simply do the squat move for a good burn.

Too little? To take this move up a notch, you can do the "donkey" squat. I saw this in a magazine and have wondered why it was named after a donkey. I have a dear friend who owns four gorgeous donkeys. (OK, they own her if you want to know the truth.) So I asked her why she thought it was named after donkeys. She guessed that it mirrors the motion right before they kick backwards. Personally, I think it is because these squats require determination that borders on stubbornness!

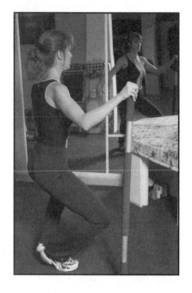

Don't start off with these, but do try to work up to them. What I like about them is that they also work your calves. I encourage you to stand next to a wall or use a pole for assistance. Start by standing with your feet in a "V" position (heels together and toes out). Raise up your heels now so that you are balancing on your toes. Now, take the squat down, moving your knees to the side (this works a different part of the glute and quad), making another "V" shape. Go as far down as you can, and come back up. Make sure to breathe on the way up, as you will need it! Do not overdo it, and stop if you experience pain.

Calves

Speaking of your calves, they need to be worked, too. A simple yet very effective way to work them is a calf raise.

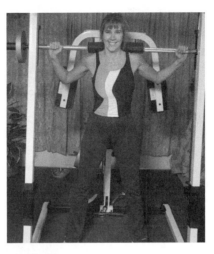

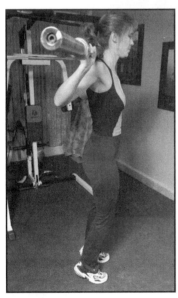

You can use the machine as indicated here or hold hand weights. Just make sure that you squeeze and hold at the top before you lower your heels back down. Slow and controlled is the key here. Do not forget to lift the toes up (just the opposite movement) to work the front of your calf, which is used to walk or hike.

NOTE: After you finish this exercise, take special care as you walk! You may find your feet a bit sluggish to lift for a while, which might make you more inclined to trip.

Inner/outer thigh

The muscle on the outer part of your leg (its official name is the *illiotibula band*, or IT band) connects right into your knee. This muscle is notorious for causing knee problems. Keep it strong with these exercises. The first one incorporates a yoga hold, which will work your core muscles, too.

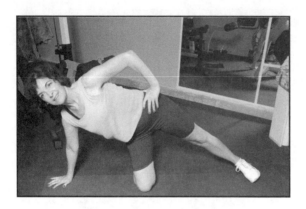

You start off by kneeling on the floor and keeping your upper body straight. Take one leg out to the side, and put your opposite hand down to the floor (left leg out and right hand down). Your leg, hip, and hand should create a straight line. You and your feet are facing forward. Lift the stretched-out leg up for a lift, and lower it down slowly. Breathe out on the lift. When you are done with your set, keep that leg stretched out and reach the same arm (left leg, left arm) up over your head for a good stretch.

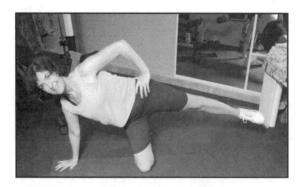

Another great option is to toss a weighted ball from side to side. Your legs are wide apart, and your toes are facing forward. The movement comes from the inner/outer leg…side to side. Take the ball, and reach down toward your right foot, then your left foot. It's a smooth move between your feet. You will feel this in the inner leg, but the outer leg is also working. Most gyms have inner and outer thigh machines that really concentrate on the muscle. Just follow the diagrams.

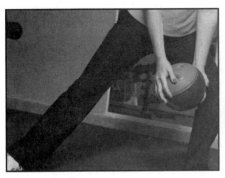 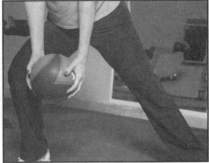

Biceps

I like to change the traditional bicep curl up a bit by holding the weights like a hammer.

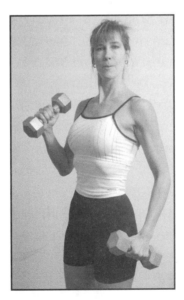

The weights are facing your body rather than facing up, like you have a hammer in each hand. With the weights in each hand and to your side, lift one up at a time, slowly lowering while the other arm comes up.

Remember to control your breathing.

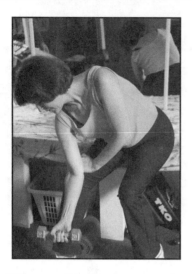 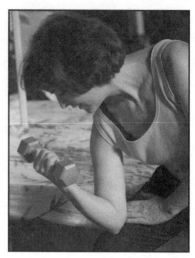

You can also do one-armed curls that really isolate the bicep. Sit down, and put your left hand on your right knee. Place your right elbow on top of your left hand. With your weight in hand and arm extended down, curl it up toward you. Never lock the elbow while lowering the weight. Breathe out on the curl up.

You can isolate the muscle even further by standing up against a wall where your triceps (back of your arm) and your back are pressed against the wall. You have just eliminated any support for these muscles to give the bicep, so the bicep is on its own. Curl with both hands together, never locking the elbows. You may need to drop your weight down on these because they are tough!

You can also do a curl without any weights, as Tim is demonstrating. When you concentrate on the movement and breathe correctly, you can still get an effective workout.

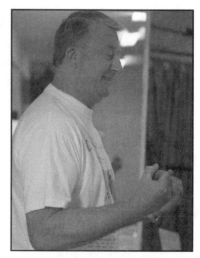

Triceps

As I just mentioned, the back of the arm is the triceps. To work these, stand up and hold a hand weight with both hands. Place it over your head, and bend your arms behind your head, keeping your elbows as close together as possible. You press the weight up over your head and lower it back down. Again, keep those elbows tight and together.

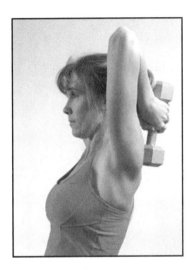 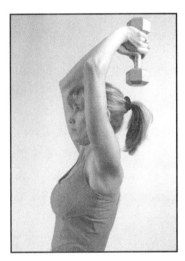

You can simply do dips without any weight involved. Use a bench or a step, and place your hands on it facing your bottom (gripping the bench or step with your palms for stability). The further you take your legs out, the harder the workload on your triceps. Want an additional burn? Lift one leg up while you dip.

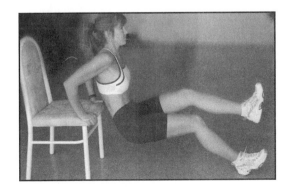

Dip down, and press yourself back up. Breathe on the way up, which is the push. Trust me, you will feel those triceps engaged. Gyms have equipment that does the same thing if you prefer a machine.

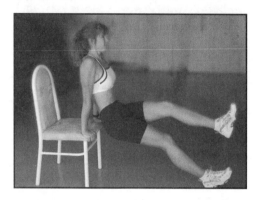

Shoulders and deltoids

Ever pour water out of a pitcher? If you have, this exercise will make sense to you. Start off facing forward and bend/hinge from the hip.

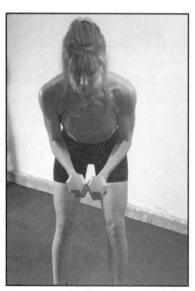

Bring the hand weights together in front of you. Keep your arms at a 90-degree angle throughout the exercise. Only the wrists change to allow you to pour the water out of your weights as if they were pitchers.

Keep your head aligned with your spine, which means you are looking down at the ground, not at yourself in the mirror or twisting your head to look at your neighbor. Go nice and easy, breathing out as you lift.

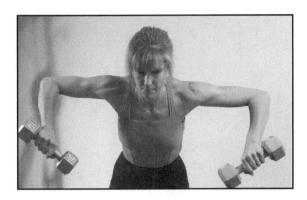

I like the "pouring water" exercise because it works your shoulders *and* your deltoids. However, if you would like to isolate each, a traditional shoulder press (overhead), followed by a side or front lift, would work. Watch the weight on these and make sure they are not too heavy. Also make sure that you don't lift too high. Never go above a straight line with your shoulder (should be even with your shoulder).

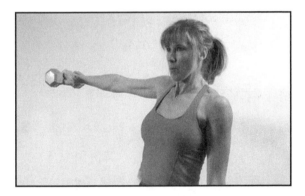

You can lift both arms together, or you can lift one at a time. Do whichever works best for you. I find that one arm at a time prevents arching the back or swaying too much.

To make the press or side lift more difficult, add a resistance ball. Place one knee on the ball just to add a little instability. Conduct the exercise as normal, except now you will have to work harder with your core muscles engaged.

Pecs

The bench press is a standard exercise for your pecs, because it sure works. You can perform a press on a bench machine or with a weighted bar. You can even use hand weights and lie on the floor. It is a very versatile exercise.

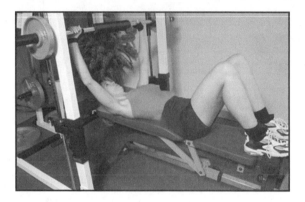

In this picture we've added a resistance ball that makes the movement more difficult. In either case, keep your head looking up, and don't dip your elbows below your body. In the raised position your arms and chest should form a big oval, never locking the elbows.

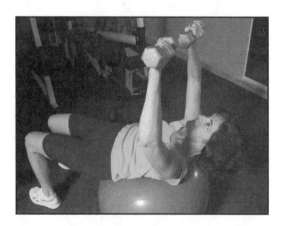

Remember to squeeze the pec muscles together and make them—not the elbow joints—do the work.

If you would like to weave another option into the variety of presses, try a "butterfly." This machine brings your arms together in front of you. You squeeze the arms together, working the pecs.

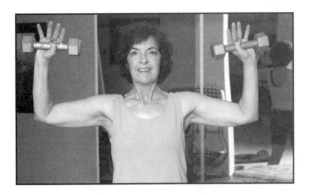

Be careful on the return (opening arms back up) as some machines allow you to go too far back, and you can strain your shoulder and/or rotator cuff. I prefer letting one arm go back at a time and slowly helping the other return. Always sit with your face and feet forward. Do not arch your back.

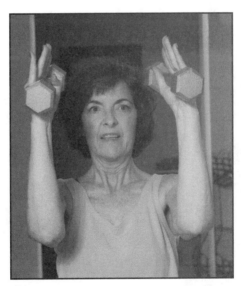

And let's not forget the good old standby: push-ups! See chapter seven for some adaptations that might work for you.

Lats and rhomboids

If you live near a lake, you may already know how great rowing is for your body. It utilizes so many muscles; it's almost a complete body workout by itself. But the muscles it really works are your lats and rhomboids. We can simulate this with a machine or with hand weights.

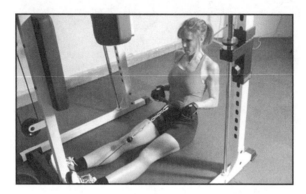

If you are on a machine, lean back just a bit with your legs straight out in front of you (without locking the knees). Pull the weight toward you, and allow your elbows to go past your torso. Bring them as far back as you can, and then let them come forward. Do not move your upper body or lock the knees. Let your arms do the work.

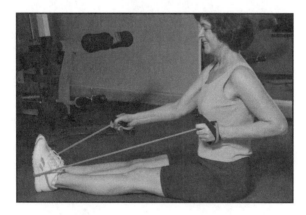

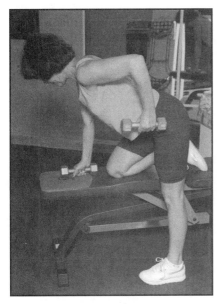

If you are using hand weights, you can stand up, bend over, and lift one arm at a time behind you. Or if you are using bands, you can sit on the floor and wrap the band around your feet and pull behind you—squeeze your shoulder blades together as you try to get your elbows to touch behind you. We will be forever pulling things such as chairs and moving furniture and boxes, so this is a great one to incorporate into your routine.

A similar move that will challenge your rhomboids a bit more is the "swimming on a ball" exercise. Place your tummy on a resistance ball with a weight in each hand. Your legs are behind you either bent or straight.

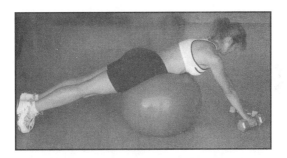

Keep your head and neck aligned with your spine (looking at the floor). Start off with your hands out in front, over your head (like a Superman pose), and then bring them down to your side. It is similar to the breaststroke…as if you are pushing water away. The difference is that you have hand weights instead of water resistance.

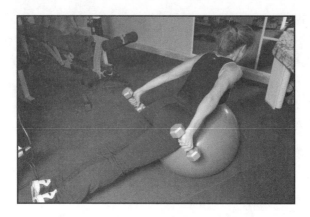

Pull-down machines provide yet another opportunity to work these back muscles. Want to change it up? Kneel down on one knee and pull down. This gives you a greater reach, working the muscle farther down the back.

Erector spinae (back)

If you have ever suffered back pain in your life, then you would benefit from keeping this muscle strong. Without it, we really can't do anything. I know folks who are literally bedridden when their backs go out on them. An ounce of prevention can save you a world of hurt.

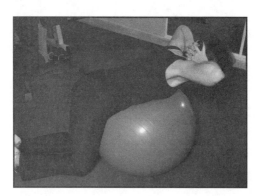

I am fond of the resistance ball here, because it offers support for the opposing muscle, the abs. Having a ball also helps this exercise really work the lower back.

Place your tummy on the resistance ball with your legs bent, knees on the floor. Your head and neck are aligned with your spine. You keep your head looking at the floor throughout the movement. Place your hands behind your head, and lift yourself up using the lower back. This is basically the complete opposite of a sit-up. Your muscles will be warm, but you should not feel any pain. Work within your range of motion. The stronger your lower back gets, the higher you will be able to lift your torso.

If this is too much to start with, take it to the floor. Lie face down. Your legs will be straight behind you. Again, keep your head and neck aligned with your spine, face to the floor. Bring your hands around, and place them under your forehead.

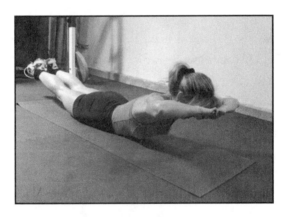

Lift your head and both your feet in one fluid motion. Don't hold it up there, but simply lower it back down. Lift up and lower. You will feel the lower back working.

Abs and obliques

If you want to have a healthy back, then you will need to work your abs. Many backaches actually come from weak abs. I have some outstanding workouts that will build abdominal strength.

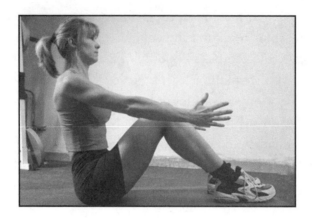

Sit up nice and tall on the floor with your knees bent. Bring your arms out in front of you, and keep them there. Lean back until the small of your back touches the floor. Gravity will want to pull you down, but sit back up.

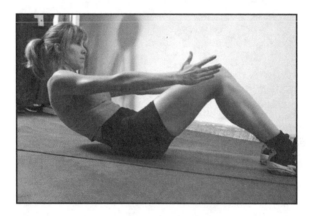

Most sit-ups reverse the movement, but this one really challenges the abs. They are pulling your weight back up. After you do enough reps, lean back and hold the position. Add a rotation, elbow side to side, to work the obliques. Ooh, baby! This will work you. Never hold your breath. Keep breathing!

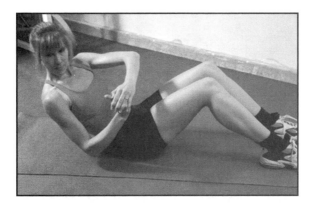

Another great way to work both the abs and your obliques (love handles) is bicycling. You don't even need a bike for this one. Lie on your back, face up, and bring your right knee to your left elbow, then left knee to right elbow. The higher your legs, the easier this will be. The lower your legs, the more your abs are required to hold the position. Pick a level that works for you. This may get your heart rate going, as it is a quick movement.

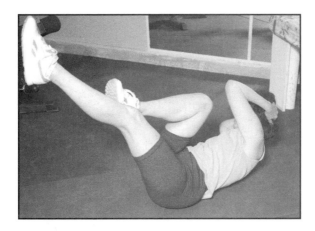

If this all sounds too fancy for you, the basic sit-up is still effective. Remember to keep your head looking up. Always have space between your chin and your chest. Make a fist, and you should be able to fit it between your chin and chest. This prevents neck strain.

PHYSICAL FITNESS

You have just learned a bunch of ways to build strength and exercise for your stage of life. I encourage you to give them a try. Don't feel bad if you forget and have to keep looking back at the pictures. It takes time to create new habits. One of my clients kept forgetting how to breathe right for months. One day, it just clicked for him. Don't expect too much of yourself. We are only human!

Be sure to be safe now so that you can enjoy the other chapters of this book designed for the next two stages of life. Things will continue to change, but the good news is that you will be ready for it! Get physical and stay active.

Chapter Seven

Focused Fitness for Fifty-Six- to Sixty-Five-Year-Olds

By this stage of life, you have seen a lot of change. Thirty years ago may not feel that long ago to you, but things have certainly changed. Here is what a thirty-year difference can do:[1]

1975	2005
KEG	EKG
Acid rock	Acid reflux
Moving to CA because it's "cool"	Moving to CA because it's warm
Trying to look like Liz Taylor	Trying NOT to look like Liz Taylor
Hoping for a BMW	Hoping for a BM
Going to a new, "hip" joint	Receiving a new hip
Rolling Stones	Kidney stones
Passing the driver's test	Passing the vision test

OK, you get the picture! You are not as young as you once were, but you can be forever young at heart. No one can take that away from you. The aging process is what it is, and you now understand what role you can play in your future health. If you truly want to be forever young, then you must take care of yourself.

Congratulations on starting wherever you are today. I am proud of you. No matter what your life looked like up until this point, you begin to improve the quantity and the quality of your life by exercising. If you haven't read chapter five, I encourage you to review the basics before you develop your own program. It provides a great foundation upon which to build.

STAGES OF LIFE

At this stage of life (fifty-six to sixty-five years old), you may or may not be retired. Folks in our country seem to be working until later in life these days, with the average age of retirement approaching sixty-seven.[2] Most likely, your children are all grown, and you have had the opportunity to do some traveling or take up new or favorite pursuits.

My in-laws are gone for a month at a time filling up the pages of their passports. Prior to retirement, they worked hard either raising their family or paying off debt. Extensive travel was not an option due to work and financial constraints. So when they had plenty of time and some extra money, they embarked on a self-focused phase. This is very typical and healthy, especially since they were coming out of strapped financial years.

These years are paramount for creating endurance.

However, if this is you, you may eventually find yourself tired of the travel and missing your home. If your friends cannot travel with you, you may also start to feel disconnected. At some point, you will probably choose to be home more often.

Research is showing that more and more folks in your age bracket are raising their grandchildren either part time or full time. A generation with a high divorce rate is affecting everyone.

No matter what your stage, these years are very important for your long-term health. You must make the time to care for yourself regardless of your situation.

This chapter is dedicated to you fifty-six- to sixty-five-year-olds. Together, we will customize an exercise program that will fit into your full life without hurting you. These are the years that are paramount to creating endurance in order to go the distance with good health. Look up *endurance* in a thesaurus, and you will find words such as *stamina*, *staying power*, and *survival*. Want a healthy future? Endurance is critical.

Rather than pushing your body harder during these years, I encourage you to work it *smarter*. You don't have to sacrifice your performance; in fact, you might see an improvement. My brother has beaten me at tennis my entire life. Even as I got stronger and more aggressive at the game, he always seemed to pull it off, usually without too much exertion. As I got older, I began to incorporate endurance training into my weekly schedule. I began to see that I did not have to run *harder* but more efficiently. The last time my brother and I played, I won. I finally got him at his own game. I did not run around the court but strategically placed the ball. This is your season to do the same.

Be strategic. Put your exercise time (both cardio and resistance training) on your calendar just as you would any other appointment.

SCHEDULE YOUR CARDIOVASCULAR EXERCISE

These years are the time for you to adapt programs to match your lifestyle and stage of life. In the chart below, the "intensity" column refers back to the Workout Intensity Chart on page 54. See what works for you and your lifestyle—but please do something.

You may have something else you like to do, and that is great. These are just suggestions that will help you get enough cardiovascular exercise in, and at the right intensity, so that you experience a health benefit without harming yourself. Remember, you are striving for long-term health here!

Whatever you select as your exercise(s), I encourage you to put it on your calendar. Work everything else around your workout schedule. You probably have more flexibility in your schedule now, so use it to your advantage. Schedule doctor's appointments and social events at times that do not conflict with your exercise.

Most seasoned veteran classes are every Monday, Wednesday, and Friday at the same time for that reason. You can count on it. Allow only emergencies and rare situations to interfere. This is *your* health we are talking about; treat it with respect.

Chart 7.1—Exercise Programs for Fifty-Six- to Sixty-Five-Year-Olds

Exercise	Frequency	Intensity
Walking	3–5 times a week	Level 7–$8\frac{1}{2}$ (Try to keep a fast pace and add some hills.)
Jogging on a treadmill	3–5 times a week	Level 7–$8\frac{1}{2}$ (Concentrate on consistency of breathing, not so much heavy breathing.)
Indoor cycling	3 times a week	Level $6\frac{1}{2}$–$8\frac{1}{2}$ (Strive for a steady heart rate or breathing pattern.)
Outdoor cycling	3–5 times a week	Level $6\frac{1}{2}$–$8\frac{1}{2}$ (Go for the distance and relatively flat course with some rolling hills.)
Swimming	3–5 times a week	Level $6\frac{1}{2}$–$7\frac{1}{2}$ (Keep smooth strokes, and don't worry about speed.)
Aqua class	3–5 times a week	Level 7–$8\frac{1}{2}$ (Follow the instructor, but always work at your pace.)
Seasoned veterans class	3 times a week	Level 7–$8\frac{1}{2}$ (Only go higher if you have been exercising for months or years.)
Circuit class	3 times a week	Level 7–$8\frac{1}{2}$ (Keep most of your workload at a solid pace. Go higher if you are physically able—but for a brief period only.)
Yoga and/or Pilates	3–5 times a week	Level 6–7

Time	Tips for Your Stage
20 minutes at level 8; 30 minutes total	Walking is still the best exercise out there because it is low impact. Make sure you are working out, not strolling. Incorporate hills.
20 minutes at level 8; 30 minutes total	If you already jog, this is the perfect option. If you are a walker, you can always weave in a little jog now and then. Treadmills are easy on the joints and allow you to set your pace and keep it.
1 hour	Most classes are one hour in length. The climbing and endurance classes may work best. NOTE: Cycle shorts or gel seats help with comfort. Always get your bike fitted properly.
At least 30 minutes	If you're a cyclist, you love being outside. But this is a great way to exercise even for the novice cyclist. Map out safe routes you are familiar with. Wear your helmet, and bring plenty of water.
20–30 minutes	Dive in, swim your laps, and get out. It's a fast, effective workout as it really builds your upper body strength.
1 hour	These classes are designed to work using the water as resistance, so you can get both cardio and muscle work in—all without impact.
1 hour	These classes are designed to be low impact. Besides being a great workout, they are typically fun and provide a social outlet. Look for alternative moves if you need them for aches and pains.
1 hour	These classes, like the seasoned veterans classes, combine cardio with sculpting. They are a great way to get both cardio and resistance training in. This is individualized, because you pick your own weight level. Don't compete with others. This is your workout.
1 hour	Yoga and Pilates both work your core muscles and flexibility. Try a class or work one-on-one with a trainer. Remember to breathe properly, which is important for both of these. Start off with beginner moves, and work your way up.

Exercise	Frequency	Intensity
Tennis	3–5 times a week	Level 7–8$\frac{1}{2}$
Jumping rope	3–5 times a week	Level 8–8$\frac{1}{2}$ (Watch your heart rate and monitor how you feel. Your heart rate can increase quickly. Jump rope at this intensity level only if you have practiced before.)
Elliptical machine	3–5 times a week	Level 7–8$\frac{1}{2}$ (Steady is the name of the game here. Be smooth yet effective.)
Senior sports teams	1–3 times a week	Level 6–7$\frac{1}{2}$ (Don't try to beat the twenty-year-olds. Enjoy fellowship with your generation.)
Hiking, canoeing, etc.	1–3 times a week	Level 6–7$\frac{1}{2}$ (Go for enjoyment)
Bowling	1–3 times a week	Level 5–7
Golf	3–5 times a week	Level 5–7

Exercise program log

On page 138 is a chart that may help you schedule and track your cardiovascular workouts. I encourage you to use it, especially if you have trouble getting your cardio workouts in each week. This will act as somewhat of an accountability partner or success record. Some people love cardio and get plenty of activity in each week. Others have to work at it. Regardless of what type you are, this program log helps you plan your exercise and protect it.

Time	Tips for Your Stage
At least 30 minutes	Most matches are $1\frac{1}{2}$–2 hours in length. Doubles provides a good workout without as much running. This game is much more strategic and requires smart playing.
8–15 minutes	Eight minutes is an eternity with a jump rope, and it may take you a lot of practice to build up to it. This is an intensive workout that maximizes time. Be easy on your joints, and don't jump hard; rather, be smooth and light on your feet. "Float like a butterfly and sting like a bee," as Muhammad Ali said.
20 minutes at level 8; 30 minutes total	Another indoor option that is easy on the joints. Keep your hands on the equipment at all times. Be careful stepping off as your balance may be off.
At least 30 minutes	These are fun activities that usually are not too intense, especially if they are played for fun. Variety is the key, so get other exercise in if possible.
At least 30 minutes	Outdoor activities are a superb way to enjoy your family and get exercise. You probably have good flexibility, so get out in God's country!
1 hour	Bowling is not high on the cardio scale, but it can be if you keep moving. Engage your arms, and use your legs. Avoid smoky bowling alleys if possible.
At least 1 hour	Golf is not a very aerobic activity, but it involves walking, which can be. Don't use a cart, but walk rapidly.

NOTE: On the log, "mode" refers to how you worked out. Examples are listed above. "Intensity" is the level of workload. Put the level that you feel the majority of your workout was spent. I recommend you make copies of this form and use it as needed. Others may prefer to log their cardio exercise in their day planner. Do whatever works for you!

Chart 7.2—Exercise Program Log

DAY/DATE	MODE	TIME	INTENSITY	NOTES
Monday				
Tuesday				
Wednesday				
Thursday				
Friday				
Saturday				
Sunday				
Monday				
Tuesday				
Wednesday				
Thursday				
Friday				
Saturday				
Sunday				
Monday				
Tuesday				
Wednesday				
Thursday				
Friday				
Saturday				
Sunday				
Monday				
Tuesday				
Wednesday				
Thursday				
Friday				
Saturday				
Sunday				

Monday				
Tuesday				
Wednesday				
Thursday				
Friday				
Saturday				
Sunday				
Monday				
Tuesday				
Wednesday				
Thursday				
Friday				
Saturday				
Sunday				
Monday				
Tuesday				
Wednesday				
Thursday				
Friday				
Saturday				
Sunday				

Adapting is important

No matter what type of exercise you choose, remember to work at your own level and adapt accordingly. Most fitness classes will offer several levels of intensity, allowing you to pick the workout that is right for you. On pages 140–143 are some ways for you to adapt the intensity level of the exercises I have recommended for your cardio workout.

Chart 7.3—Customize Your Intensity Level (Ages Fifty-Six to Sixty-Five)

EXERCISE	LOW INTENSITY (Levels 1–4)	MEDIUM INTENSITY (Levels 5–7)
Walking	Flat, short course (1–3 miles)	Longer course or rolling hills (3–5 miles)
Jogging on a treadmill	Keep the grade at 0, and alternate power walking with a slight jog for 1–3 miles.	Increase the grade to 5 and power walk, swinging arms on sides.
Indoor cycling	Endurance class or beginner	Climbing/strength or intermediate
Outdoor cycling	Flat, short course (8–10 miles)	Longer course with rolling hills (10–15 miles)
Swimming	Indoor pool laps (10 laps)	Indoor pool laps (20 laps)
Aqua class	Keep arms down.	Raise arms up.
Seasoned veterans class	Arms down, legs close together, side steps, no impact	Arms up, legs farther apart, higher lifts
Circuit class	No weights or very light weights, no impact	Light to medium weights, legs farther apart
Yoga and/or Pilates	Beginner stretches	Moves that require holding
Tennis	Mixed doubles	Doubles
Jumping rope	Soft and easy steps over the rope; slow and controlled. Or simulate the movement without the rope.	Swing the legs a bit more as you step over the rope.
Elliptical machine	Slow cadence without arms. Hold on to side if necessary.	Medium cadence with arms swinging
Senior sports teams	Sports that involve rotation of players so you get to rest	Sports that require more involvement

HIGH INTENSITY (Levels 8–10)	NOTES
Longer course or hills (5–8 miles)	Make sure to have supportive shoes. Using your arms will increase the intensity. Adding hand weights takes it up even more.
Increase the grade to 8 or higher. You can also keep it flat but walk faster.	Try a 12-minute mile pace, and see how you do. You can increase or decrease the speed at any time. Use the handgrips if needed for support. Be careful stepping off.
All-terrain or difficult	Even at level 3, you can still control your own gear. Sit down instead of standing up. Keep pedaling, and you will get a good workout regardless.
Longer course with hills (15–50 miles)	Know your route, and stick to cycle lanes to avoid any accidents. Wear your helmet!
Indoor pool laps (30 or more)	You can add water weights to your arms and legs to increase the workload.
Add water weights for additional resistance.	Follow the instructor. Be careful getting in and out of the pool area.
Arms up, legs farther apart, and add impact (full jumping jacks)	Don't go too high too fast. The good news is that you can take it down any time you need to. Every day is different. Don't expect to perform at the same level all the time.
Medium to heavier weights, add impact	If you concentrate on the muscle you want to work, you can still get some benefit without the weight. Be safe.
Moves that have extra resistance and require balance	Breathing is essential. Don't hold your breath! Follow the instructor or trainer.
Singles	Be strategic with your play. Keep moving.
Add a hop over the rope, and use both legs if it is not too much impact.	Really engage the arms/wrists with or without the rope.
Faster cadence with arms swinging	Set the machine for a certain time rather than going for speed.
Sports that have fewer players	Pick one that you like, and stick to it.

EXERCISE	LOW INTENSITY (Levels 1–4)	MEDIUM INTENSITY (Levels 5–7)
Hiking, canoeing, etc.	1–5 miles, flat and calm	6–10 miles, flat and calm
Bowling	Recreational play only	Low-level teams
Golf	Recreational practice at driving ranges or putt-putt golf	9 holes

Here Tim is showing a simple way to adapt the basic jumping jack and make it low impact. Be creative. Make it work for you!

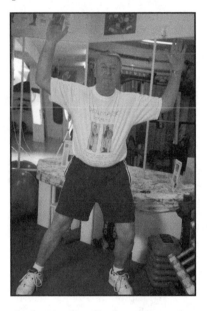

Weight-Bearing Training

As I have mentioned, your exercise must also include resistance training. Even though these are your years to create endurance, you still need to work your muscles for healthy bones. You don't need to push as hard, and you may reduce your weights, but please continue to include resistance training in your routine. Remember, the stronger your muscles the healthier your bones. Eventually, our bones will start to lose mass. The bigger they are to begin with, the better off you will be.

HIGH INTENSITY (Levels 8–10)	NOTES
Add hills or rougher water.	Do your homework before embarking on outdoor activities. Heed the ratings systems and come prepared. Never go alone.
More competitive teams	Watch and protect your wrists. Don't go too heavy with the ball.
18 holes	Walk fast between holes, and practice that swing!

Which weight is right for you?

If you lifted weights regularly in your earlier years, you have built up strong muscles and bones. You may find, however, that you have had to reduce your weights as you have aged. Don't compare yourself to another time in life; you will only frustrate yourself. Use a weight that is difficult enough to push you but not hurt you.

The best way to find a weight that is right for you is to spend time evaluating each muscle and trying a variety of weights. For example, a woman may start off with only three-pound hand weights for her bicep curl. She should soon be able to increase this to five or six pounds, which is plenty for her goals of endurance. Men are tradi-tionally stronger because they have more testosterone and more mus-cle fibers. They should be able to lift six- to eight-pound hand weights to start and build from there. Men get stronger quicker, but they should also be careful of overdoing it. Remember, you are working toward long-term health.

Partner up

If you are lifting weights outside of the seasoned veterans class, lift with a buddy, even if you are using the machines. In fact, I really don't see the need for you to use free weights at this stage of the game unless it has been a part of your life for a very long time. If you are accus-tomed to free weights, then use them, but I still encourage you to have a partner. Partners are important for exercises that could harm you, such as the bench press. People have been severely hurt by the bar when they have lost control of it. Be safe, or you could find yourself in trouble. The machines offer a very good workout but are safer over-all (if you follow the instructions).

If you work out at a club or fitness center, do not compare your-self to anyone else. No one is the same. We are different ages with dif-ferent fitness levels and different goals. Remember, small steps for you will do the trick! Any resistance training is better than none. If your muscles have not been worked before, they will be weak. This is a fact. But the exciting news is that your body will respond quickly. Before you know it, you will increase your muscle mass and bone density, both of which are important.

Caution

During any exercise, whether cardiovascular or weight lifting, if you experience pain, stop! Your body is telling you something. It is better to listen up front to your body's whisper than experience it screaming at you later. A little prevention will help you stay at it longer. Pain is often an indicator of too much, too soon.

If you feel pain when doing cardio exercise (muscle pain, not breathing complications), simply reduce your impact, lower your arms, or walk in place. With weight lifting, lower the amount of weights until you eventually build yourself up to a heavier weight. If at any time you experience symptoms remotely close to a heart attack, seek medical attention immediately.

It's better to listen to your body's whisper than its scream.

This does not mean you should never feel anything uncomfort-able. If you are embarking on a new fitness program, you *will* feel it. You will experience some soreness and muscle fatigue. This is part of the process. If you follow the guidelines in this book, however, such discomfort should be minimal. But nonetheless, it is par for the course when starting a new workout routine.

I mentioned earlier that I highly suggest you seek the counsel of a physician before you start your new program. I can't emphasize this enough, especially if you are overweight or have been living a sedentary lifestyle. If you have a family history of heart disease or other restrictive ailments, you definitely need to get a checkup and overall physical before you begin. Better to be safe than sorry!

Endurance log

I suggest you log your resistance training, as you did with your cardio exercise. This chart will ensure that you don't forget a muscle. I spend every day training people, and I still use this log for myself.

Chart 7.4—Weight-Bearing Exercise Log

Muscle	Mode	Seat/ Settings	Weight/ Reps #1	Weight/ Reps #2	Weight/ Reps #3	Stretch?
Quads						
Hamstrings						
Glutes						
Calves						
Inner thigh						
Outer thigh						
Forearms, hands						
Biceps						
Triceps						
Shoulders						
Deltoids						
Pecs						
Lats/ rhomboids						
Erector spinae						
Abs						
Obliques						

Weight-lifting Exercises for Specific Muscle Groups

The following exercises use a combination of floor work, free weights, and exercise machines. Each one works a major muscle.

Quads, hamstrings, and glutes

Lunges are among my favorite exercises, because they work three muscle groups at once (quads, hamstrings, and glutes) as well as challenging our core muscles. However, if done incorrectly, lunges can hurt. Pay attention to your form at all times. NOTE: If you have severe knee damage, such as bone on bone, use a leg machine instead.

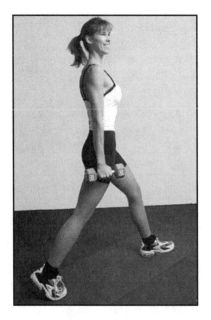

The starting position for a lunge is putting one leg forward and one leg back. Most people make the mistake of not putting their back leg far enough behind them. Spread your legs apart. Stand up straight. The movement comes from your back knee, not the front. The front knee will remain stable, and you should be able to see your toes throughout the movement.

Lower your back leg down, and bring it back up. Your head, spine, and back knee are aligned when you go down (as if a pole is running through your body). If these are too unstable for you, add a pole or hold on to a wall for support. You can also change lunges up by stepping forward instead of back or walking the length of a room. I encourage you to master the basic lunge first before taking on more difficult versions. The basic lunge is a phenomenal leg workout.

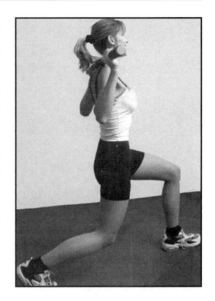

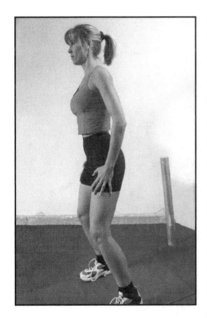

Another great option for your legs is a squat. This mirrors a movement we will do the rest of our lives: sitting down and getting up. Your feet should be shoulder-width apart with your feet facing forward. Push your glute out behind you as if you are trying to sit on a chair. As soon as you get close to the chair (no more than a 90-degree angle), come back up. I like to push my arms out in front of me for counter balance. It also helps remind you to push out behind. Your knees should never go forward, and you should be able to see your toes. Keep your heels flat on the floor the whole time.

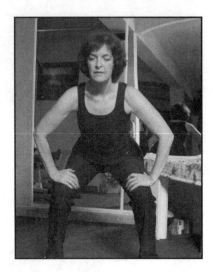

You can change up this simple move and make it a bit more difficult by adding a side lift with your squat. Just as you are coming back up, lift one leg to your side, using your hip and glute. Go back to the standing position, squat again, and then lift the other leg up. This is an awesome workout for your hip abductors, outer thigh, and inner thigh, along with the other leg muscles.

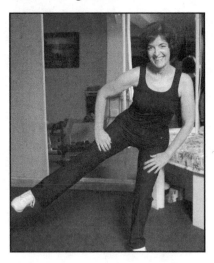

Calves

We don't want to forget your calves. Although they are recruited for some of the leg exercises mentioned, you should still concentrate solely on them once in a while.

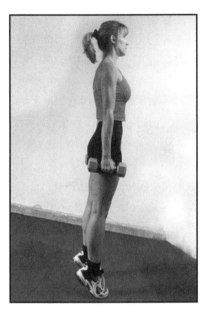

Get some light hand weights to hold, one in each hand. Raise your heels up, and stand on your toes. Hold and squeeze this for a few seconds before you lower your heels. Slow and controlled is the key here. Then lift your toes up (just the opposite movement) to work the front of your calf, which is used to walk or hike.

NOTE: After you finish this exercise, take special care as you walk! You may find your feet a bit sluggish to lift for a while, which might make you more inclined to trip.

You can change this move up by adding a stool or step. Place the balls of your feet on the step, and lower your heels down as far as they will go. This is a wonderful stretch. Then raise the heels up as high as you can go. Pause at the top before lowering again. You can add hand weights to make it harder, and you can use a pole or wall for stability.

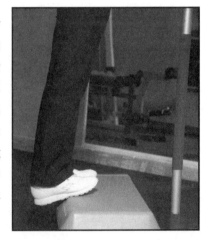

Inner/outer thigh

Besides the squat and side lift move, you can also work your inner and outer thigh with a Pilates ring. You can purchase one at any sporting goods store or Barnes and Noble bookstore. It is typically green with black handles, and it comes with a little video to give you ideas on how to use it. This move works both the outer (official name is the illiotibula band, or IT band) and your inner thigh at the same time.

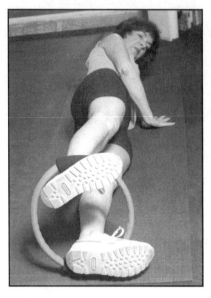

Start off by lying on your side. Your head, hip, and ankles should be in a straight line. Place your feet into the ring with your top leg holding the ring up and the bottom leg holding the ring down. This is an opposing muscle workout. Each muscle is trying to do something different: one wants to lift up and the other is holding it down. By doing this, you are working both muscles. Each squeeze is a count of one. Remember to breathe and keep one foot on the ground. If you don't have access to a ring, then refer to the previous chapter for a description of floor side lifts.

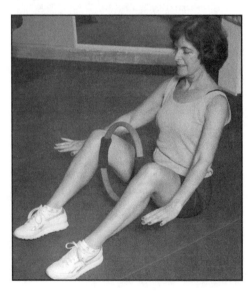

You can use the green ring to work your inner thighs only by sitting up with your legs bent in front of you. Place the ring between your knees and squeeze it together. You can also stand and do the same movement. Each squeeze is a count of one.

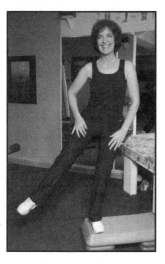

The outer thigh can be worked with a step. The higher the risers, the more difficult the move, so keep it low. Stand to the side of the step. Step one foot up onto the step while lifting the other leg up to your side, using your hip abductors again. Step back down, and do several reps on each leg. These are great for building strong hips and strengthening your core muscles, not to mention your coordination. Watch your step.

Biceps

To work your biceps, a weighted bar is a nice option. You can even use a broomstick if you are a beginner. The starting position is standing upright with your legs shoulder-width apart, knees soft, and feet forward. Hold the bar with your wrists facing up and arms extended down toward your legs without locking the elbows.

Curl the bar up toward you as you breathe out. Breathe in as you lower it again, and repeat.

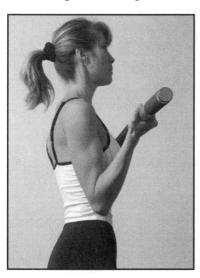

Do not lean with your back or swing. If you find yourself moving a lot as you lift, you probably have too much weight. Reduce your weight so that the arms, not the back, are doing the work. Never lock the elbows while lowering the weight, and don't lock your knees either. Breathe out on the curl up.

You can change up the bicep curl by using handheld weights and having your wrists facing toward your body, arms by your side. This is called a "hammer curl" as it simulates hammering a nail. Alternate arms or lift together, but the same rules apply: breathe out on the up.

Triceps

To work the opposite muscle of your biceps, which is the triceps, a great option is what I call the "triceps pushback." You'll need hand weights in each hand.

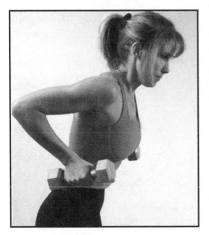

Stand with your feet shoulder-width apart and hinge forward from your hip. You should be looking down at the floor. Now, raise your elbows up high behind you on each side. Hinging from the elbow and not moving the back part of the arm, push your hands back behind you.

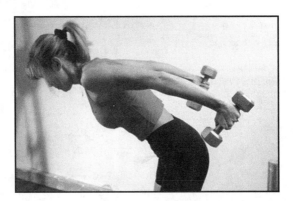

Breathe out as you push back, and breathe in when you bring them back to the starting position. Keep the elbows high, head down, and don't swing the arm loosely. These are tough!

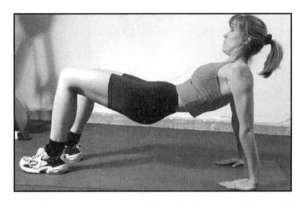

You can work the triceps on the floor as well. Sit down on the floor with your hands/fingers facing your glute (awkward at first). Your knees are bent. Using your triceps, lift your entire torso off the ground. This is like a push-up, but in reverse. Bend the arms up and down. Don't lock the elbows or move your torso. You should feel this in your triceps. Breathe out as you lift up, and breathe in as you lower, never letting your glute touch the floor.

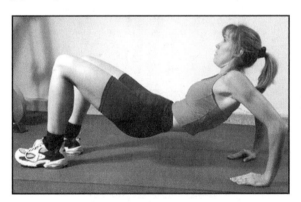

If you prefer machines, several good options exist such as the push down or pull down. Follow the directions on the machine. Also, the previous and following chapters have additional ideas you may want to consider.

Shoulders and deltoids

A great shoulder and deltoid workout for you is the front lift. Each hand has a weight. In this exercise you are facing forward with soft knees and legs shoulder-width apart. Lift one arm at a time, no higher than even with your shoulder line. Breathe out on the lift and in on the lower. Be sure you don't lock your elbows.

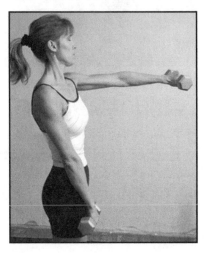

If the weight seems too much, you can use a weighted exercise ball instead. Use both hands to hold it, and follow the same steps.

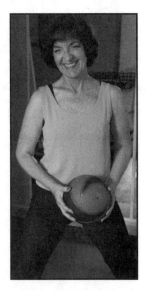

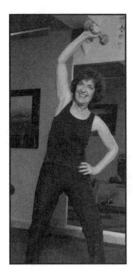

If you do not have shoulder problems, a single arm press over your head is a good workout. Rather than stand straight, lean slightly over engaging the sides of your body (obliques, or love handles). Press the weight up and over your head, breathing out. Lower it, but not too far down: basically even with your shoulder. Repeat.

For those folks with shoulder restrictions, check out the next chapter for alternatives.

Pecs

The bench press is a standard exercise for your pecs. I like the option of using handheld weights instead of the bar.

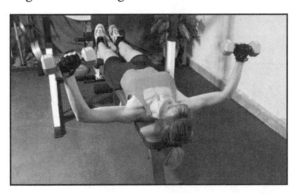

Start off by lying down with your back pressed into the bench. To help support the back, I like to bend my knees. Find whatever is most comfortable for you. You are facing up with your arms to your side, making a "U." Your elbows don't go lower than the bench. Keep them even with your shoulders. Press up with your arms, keeping the elbows slightly bent. Squeeze the pec muscles together, and make them do the pulling rather than the triceps pushing. Bring the weights together at the top. You can even have them touch out in front of you. Breathe in on the down and out on the up.

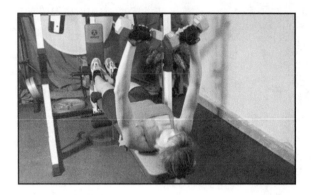

Remember to squeeze the pec muscles together and make them work, not the elbow joints. Keep looking up, and don't let the elbows go beneath the bench.

Another way to work the pec muscles is to use the Pilates ring again. This time, you have your arms out in front of you, gripping the ring with the palms of your hands, not your fingers. Squeeze the ring together as hard as you can. Each squeeze is a count of one.

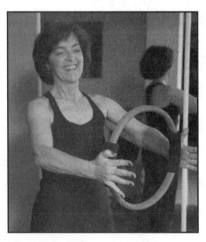

This is an isolated, contracted movement. It is amazing how quickly you will feel it. Remember that push-ups are still a tried and true pec workout as well. Look back to chapter five for pictures. Depending upon your ability, pick the level that works for you. For other ideas for the pecs that involve exercise bands, check out the next chapter as well.

Lats and rhomboids

If you have ever had a yard, you have probably mowed the grass. The movement of starting up the mower uses many muscles, but it really works your lats and rhomboids. We can mirror this with hand weights and a bench.

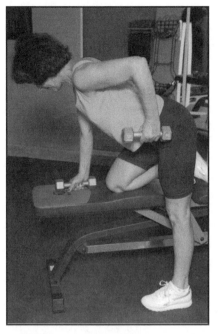

Rest your right knee and hand on a bench. Your left leg is standing on the floor, and your left hand is holding the weight. You are looking down at the bench as you pull your elbow back—just like starting a lawn mower. Don't lock your elbow on the lowering, and remember to breathe in. As you pull back, breathe out.

You can work these muscles with an exercise band, too. Hold your left arm up straight, holding one end of the band. Your other hand comes up to pull the band down and slightly back.

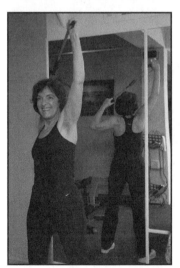

Keep your head and neck aligned with your spine (looking forward). Switch arms when you have done your reps. You will feel this in your shoulders, because they are working, too. If you have shoulder challenges, skip this one and look at the next chapter for additional ways to work these muscles with bands.

Erector spinae (back)

If you have ever suffered back pain in your life, then you would benefit from keeping this muscle strong. Without it, we really can't do anything. I know folks who are literally bedridden when their backs go out on them. An ounce of prevention can save you a world of hurt.

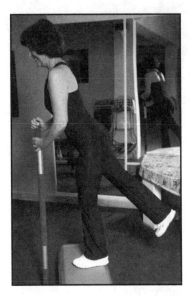

I just showed you ways to work your upper back, but now we are concentrating on the lower back. Using a low step or riser, step up with one foot all the way on the step and lift the opposite leg behind you. Keep the leg straight, and don't bend the knee. This lift is coming from the lower back and glute. You should feel these muscles engaged if you are doing it properly.

Don't try to lift too high. The key here is to have the muscle do the work we have asked it to do: lift. Breathe in as you lower and out as you lift up. Switch legs each time you step: the right leg steps up and the left leg lifts, then the left leg steps up and the right leg lifts. If you keep a pretty good pace as you step, you will get a little cardio exercise in to boot!

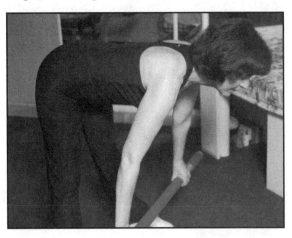

Another option for your lower back is a "dead lift." This also stretches out your hamstrings (back of the legs). NOTE: Do not do this with a heavy bar. The idea is to get movement, not strain the back. Use a four- or eight-pound weighted bar or even a broom handle. Start off standing with your feet shoulder-width apart, feet forward.

Hold the bar or broom handle with your hands, wrists facing down (knuckles up). Stand up nice and tall. Hinging from your hip, bend forward, lowering your chest.

As soon as your back starts to bend or arch, stop. You are only to go as far as your back and hamstrings will allow you. Come back up slowly, breathing in. Each time you do this, you should have a little more movement. Remember, allow the chest to lead. For additional back exercises, look at chapter six.

Abs and obliques

If you want to have a healthy back, you will need to work your abs as well. Many backaches actually come from weak abs. Here are some outstanding workouts that will help.

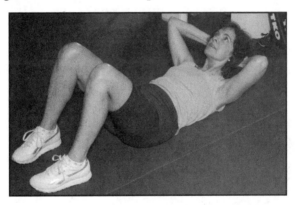

The traditional sit-up is still very effective, especially when you combine it with a rotation. Start off lying on the ground, facing up, with your knees bent. Hands are behind your neck but are not pulling on your neck. Anytime you do sit-ups, make sure you have space between your chin and chest. You should be able to fit your fist in there.

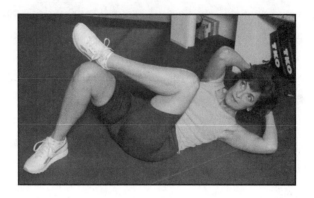

Lift your chest up and sit up. Breathe out as you go up and in as you lower back down. To engage the obliques, cross one leg over the other and bring your elbow to the opposite leg.

Your breathing pattern remains the same. Keep looking up. If you get tired and feel your stomach poofing out, stop and rest. It is better to have quality with sit-ups than quantity.

This exercise involves both the abs and obliques. You should concentrate on just the obliques now and then. A great way to target them is to stand up straight with a hand weight in each hand.

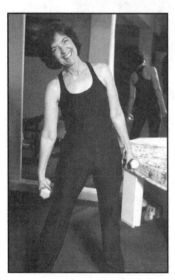

Keep your arms straight, but don't lock the elbows. Continue standing straight, and lean to the right side and then to the left. It should be a fluid movement but not super fast. If you don't want to use hand weights, you can do this same movement with a weighted ball over your head, which will also work your shoulders.

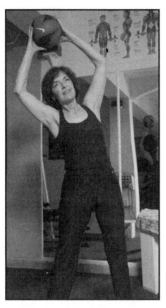

Each time you go to the right and left side is a count of one. Don't forget to breathe in as you stand up and breathe out as you lean. It's quicker breathing but still important.

FOCUSED FITNESS

Ta-da! You have just learned ways to exercise and build endurance for this stage of your life. Give them a try. Remember, it takes time to create new habits, so look back at the pictures if you need to.

Many of my clients bring printouts and workout guides with them to the gym so they can follow guidelines for an effective workout. It's the next best thing to working out with me directly.

Be safe, and never overdo it. Your body will continue to change, but the good news is that you will be ready for it! You are focused on good health for the long term.

Chapter Eight

Functional Fitness for Sixty-Six and Older

Congratulations on becoming a truly seasoned veteran. Folks in your age bracket are my inspiration.

My mom and her friends, all in their sixties, really got a kick out of the following, and I thought it might make you chuckle:

> Everything is changing. Doesn't everything seem farther away now than it used to be? It's now twice as far to the corner—and they've added a hill! Have you noticed that the bus leaves faster than it used to? Don't bother running after it. Stairs seem to be steeper than in the old days, and what is up with the smaller print in newspapers these days? No sense in asking anyone to read out loud, though. Everyone speaks in such a low tone that you can hardly hear them.
>
> The material in clothing is so skimpy, especially around the waist and the hips, that it is impossible to reach down to put your shoes on. Everyone is much younger than they used to be when you were their age. On the other hand, people your age are looking much older than you. Some folks may have aged so much that they don't even recognize you. Don't be alarmed by your own reflection…they don't make mirrors like they used to, either.

If you haven't learned this principle yet, it's time to learn it: you have to laugh at life or you'll end up crying! So what if you are not as young as you once were? You can choose to be forever young at heart.

No one can take that away from you. The aging process is what it is, and you now understand what role you can play in your future health. Chances are that you have been doing something right, so I encourage you to continue to take care of yourself.

To keep "blue skies smiling at you," look for ways to improve upon your lifestyle. We can all make improvements to our lifestyle. And no matter what your life looked like up until this point, you begin to improve the quantity and the quality of your life by exercising and eating right.

If you haven't read chapter five yet, I encourage you to do so to review the basics before you develop your own program. It provides a great foundation upon which to build.

STAGES OF LIFE

At this stage of life (sixty-six and older), you are most likely retired. Your children are all grown, and you may have so many grandchildren that you have almost lost track of their names. Well, I know you haven't, but your family has probably grown. Depending upon when you retired, you may have done some traveling—and may have even burned out on it already. Perhaps the comforts of home, such as your own bed and pillows, have become more appealing than seeing the world. Then again, you may have uprooted completely, sold your home, and gone on the road in a motor home. Rules really don't exist for folks in their retirement years. You decide what they will be...no one else.

You may have started to encounter a few more aches and pains, along with extra visits to the doctor's office. So at this stage it is especially important for your long-term health to make the time to care for yourself. Don't let travel plans be an excuse. Have workout options you can do on the road. You have started something by reading this book, and I encourage you to keep going!

This chapter is dedicated to you who are sixty-six and older. Together we will customize a healthy lifestyle that will fit into your schedule without hurting you. These are the years when we concentrate on "functional fitness," meaning that our workouts will help give you strength for things that you will always do. Mobility and flexibility are essential ingredients to continue living a healthy life well beyond your current age. Quality of life is just as important as quantity of life.

Functional fitness allows you to retain your independence as long as possible. Seasoned veterans in this age bracket don't need to worry as much about performance or strength, but should rather focus on retaining the ability to do what they want without injury.

Don't get me wrong: you can still play hard, enjoy life, and see health improvements. The body is amazing and will respond to proper exercise. But this is a different season for you, one in which the focus needs to be on longevity and safety. In our youth we may have sacrificed safety. We get by and survive. The older we get, however, the harder it is on our body to recover from abuse. Be smart.

As with any other age bracket, you still need to include both *cardio exercise* and *resistance training* in your weekly schedule. But they may look a little different for you at this stage of life than when you were younger.

Chart 8.1—Activity Ideas (Ages Sixty-Six and Older)

Exercise	Frequency	Intensity
Walking	5–7 days a week	Level 6–7 (Try to keep a fast pace, and add some hills.)
Gardening	3 days a week	Level 5–6
Indoor cycling	3 times a week	Level $6^1/_2$–$8^1/_2$ (Strive for a steady heart rate or breathing pattern.)
Outdoor cycling	3–5 times a week	Level $6^1/_2$–$8^1/_2$ (Go for the distance and a flat course.)

CUMULATIVE CARDIOVASCULAR EXERCISE

In chapter four we discussed the importance of "heart health," so I will not repeat that here. This is the time for you to adapt exercises to match your lifestyle and stage of life. Remember that cumulative exercise counts. This means that all activities throughout the day add up. Although intensity is not as important, you still want to make sure your heart is healthy.

Here are some ideas for how you can keep your heart strong. The intensity column refers to the Workout Intensity Chart on page 54. Include a variety of activities each day.

Time	Tips for Your Stage
20–30 minutes	Walking is still the best exercise out there, because it is low impact. Walk the mall, go to a park, stroll around the block—just keep moving.
1 hour	Working in the yard requires walking and a ton of bending. Use caution when lifting heavy pots or bags of soil. Make sure you lift with your legs instead of your back.
1 hour	Most classes are one hour in length. The endurance classes may work best as they involve less standing out of the saddle. NOTE: Cycle shorts or gel seats help with comfort. Carefully monitor your heart rate.
At least 30 minutes	If you are already a cyclist, you love being outside. But this is a great way to exercise even for the novice cyclist. Map out safe routes you are familiar with. Wear your helmet, and bring plenty of water.

Chart 8.1—Activity Ideas (Ages Sixty-Six and Older) cont'd

Exercise	Frequency	Intensity
Swimming	3 to 5 times a week	Level $6\frac{1}{2}$–$7\frac{1}{2}$ (Keep smooth strokes, and don't worry about speed.)
Aqua class	3–5 times a week	Level 7–$8\frac{1}{2}$ (Follow the instructor, but always work at your pace.)
Seasoned veterans class	3 times a week	Level 7–$8\frac{1}{2}$ (Only go higher if you have been exercising for several months or years.)
Sit and be fit	3 times a week	Level 6–7
Circuit class	3 times a week	Level 7–$8\frac{1}{2}$ (Keep your impact low, and use light weights.)
Tennis	3–5 times a week	Level 6–7
Yoga and/or Pilates	3–5 times a week	Level 6–7
Elliptical machine	3–5 times a week	Level 7–8 (Steady is the name of the game here. Be smooth yet effective.)
Senior sports teams	1–3 times a week	Level 6–$7\frac{1}{2}$ (Don't try to beat the twenty-year-olds. Enjoy fellowship with your generation.)
Hiking, canoeing, etc.	1–3 times a week	Level 6–$7\frac{1}{2}$ (Go for enjoyment.)

Time	Tips for Your Stage
20–30 minutes	Dive in, swim your laps, and get out. It's a fast, effective workout as it really builds your upper body strength. Bring dry clothes to change into so you don't get too chilled afterward.
1 hour	These classes are designed to work using the water as resistance, so you can get both cardio and muscle work in. Wear proper footgear to provide traction. Bring dry clothes to change into so you don't get too chilled afterward.
1 hour	These classes are designed to be low impact. Besides being a great workout, they are typically fun and provide a social outlet. Look for alternative moves if you need them because of aches and pains. Make sure to stretch afterward!
1 hour	An alternative to the seasoned veterans class, these classes are conducted from a chair for those who have knee, back, shoulder, or other challenges. They still give you a great workout and are safe for ages 66 and up.
1 hour	These classes, like the seasoned veterans class, combine cardio with sculpting. Select the lower options and easier moves. Don't compete with others. This is *your* workout.
At least 30 minutes	Most matches are $1\frac{1}{2}$–2 hours in length. Mixed doubles provides a good workout without as much running. This game is much more strategic and requires smart playing. Consider joining a 66-plus team.
1 hour	Yoga and Pilates both work your core muscles and flexibility. Try a class or work one-on-one with a trainer. Remember to breathe properly. Start off with beginner moves and work your way up.
20–30 minutes	This is another indoor option that is easy on the joints. Keep your hands on the equipment at all times. Be careful stepping off as you may have difficulty maintaining your balance.
At least 30 minutes	These are fun activities that usually are not too intense, especially if they are played for fun. Variety is the key, so get other exercise in if possible.
At least 30 minutes	Outdoor activities are a superb way to enjoy your family and get exercise. Always go prepared with emergency items and make sure someone knows where you are headed.

Exercise	Frequency	Intensity
Bowling	1–3 times a week	Level 5–7
Golf	3–5 times a week	Level 5–7
Cleaning house	1 time a week	Level 6

What else can you think of that you can count toward your cumulative exercise? Chart 8.2 below offers incentives for you.

Remember, you are striving for long-term health here! Whatever you select as your activities, I encourage you to put them on your calendar. Schedule everything else around your workout schedule. You have more flexibility with your time now, so use it to your advantage. Schedule doctor's appointments and social events at times that do not conflict with your exercise.

Most seasoned veteran classes are every Monday, Wednesday, and Friday at the same time for that reason. You can count on it. Allow only emergencies and rare situations to interfere. This is *your* health we are talking about; treat it with respect.

Chart 8.2—Calories Burned

INSTEAD OF	CALORIES BURNED	TRY	CALORIES BURNED
Taking the elevator	3	Taking the stairs	19
Using a car wash	35	Washing the car at home	104
Riding a lawn mower	88	Pushing a lawn mower	193[1]

Time	Tips for Your Stage
1 hour	Bowling is not high on the cardio scale, but it can be if you keep moving. Engage your arms and use your legs. Avoid smoky bowling alleys, if possible.
At least 1 hour	Golf is not a very aerobic activity, but it involves walking, which can be. Don't use a cart, and walk rapidly.
1 hour	This functional activity can get your heart rate up and uses muscles. Vacuum, dust, mop floors, clean blinds, etc.

Activity log

On page 170 is a chart that may help you schedule and track your cumulative activities. I encourage you to use it, especially if you have trouble getting your workouts in each week. This will act as somewhat of an accountability partner or success record.

NOTE: On the log, "mode" refers to your activity. Examples are listed above. "Intensity" is the level of workload. Put the level that you feel the majority of your activity was spent. I recommend you make copies of this form and use it as needed.

Chart 8.3—Activity Log

DAY/DATE	MODE	TIME	INTENSITY	NOTES
Monday				
Tuesday				
Wednesday				
Thursday				
Friday				
Saturday				
Sunday				
Monday				
Tuesday				
Wednesday				
Thursday				
Friday				
Saturday				
Sunday				
Monday				
Tuesday				
Wednesday				
Thursday				
Friday				
Saturday				
Sunday				
Monday				
Tuesday				
Wednesday				
Thursday				
Friday				
Saturday				
Sunday				

Adapting is the key

No matter what type of activity you choose, remember to work at your own level and adapt accordingly. Most fitness classes will offer several levels of intensity, allowing you to pick the workout that is right for you. On pages 172–173 are three levels of intensity for each of the exercises I've mentioned previously.

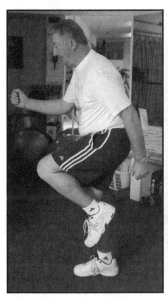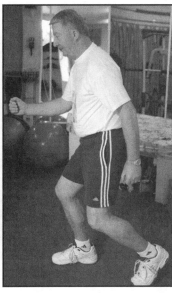

Tim is showing us here how he can lower a move to make it effective but safer for anyone with lower back pain or knee problems.

Chart 8.4—Customize Your Intensity Level (Ages Sixty-Six and Older)

Exercise	Level 1	Level 2
Walking	Flat, short course (every day)	Longer course or rolling hills (3–5 days a week)
Gardening	Stay low to the ground, with little getting up and down. Use a kneeling pad.	Move more; get up and down. Walk.
Indoor cycling	Endurance class or beginner	Climbing/strength or intermediate
Outdoor cycling	Flat, short course (3–5 miles)	Longer course with rolling hills (6–8 miles)
Swimming	Indoor pool laps (5 laps)	Indoor pool laps (10 laps)
Aqua class	Keep arms down.	Raise arms up.
Seasoned veterans class	Arms down, legs close together, side steps, no impact	Arms up, legs farther apart, higher lifts
Sit and be fit	No weights. All seated.	Light weights. Some standing.
Circuit class	No weights or very light weights, no impact (see above)	Light to medium weights, legs farther apart (some impact)
Tennis	Mixed doubles	Doubles
Yoga and/or Pilates	Beginner moves that are focused on stretching	Intermediate moves that require holding the position
Elliptical machine	Slow cadence and hold on to the railing	Medium cadence with arms swinging
Senior sports teams	Sports that involve rotation of players so you get to rest	Sports that require more involvement
Hiking, canoeing, etc.	1–3 miles, flat and calm	5–8 miles, flat and calm
Bowling	Recreational play only	Low-level teams
Golf	Recreational practice at driving ranges or miniature golf	9 holes with a cart

Level 3	Notes
Longer course or hills (3 days a week)	Make sure to have supportive shoes. Using your arms will increase the intensity. Adding hand weights takes it up even more.
Move pots and furniture yourself. Dig, shovel, and rake.	Wear your gloves and hat. Make sure you have sunscreen on. Drink plenty of water.
All-terrain or difficult	Endurance is still work. Even though you are in lower gears, the constant pace works you.
Longer course with hills (9 or more miles)	Know your route and stick to cycle lanes to avoid any accidents. If you are not comfortable clipping your feet in, don't! Make sure you have good pedals. Wear a helmet.
Indoor pool laps (20 or more laps)	This is not a race. Just keep moving.
Add water weights for additional resistance.	Follow the instructor. Be careful getting in and out of the pool area.
Arms up, legs farther apart and add impact (full jumping jacks)	Don't go too high too fast. The good news is that you can take it down any time you need to. Every day is different. Don't have expectations to perform at the same level all the time.
Medium weights. More movement as instructed.	These classes use resistance bands and other tools. Pick the ones that work best for you.
Medium to heavier weights and more impact.	If you concentrate on the muscle you want to work, you can still get some benefit without the weight. Be safe.
Singles	Be careful and listen to your body. If you are having a bad day, you can always play tomorrow.
More advanced moves that require balance	Concentrate on your core muscles (abs and back) no matter what level you work.
Faster cadence with arms swinging	Set the machine for a certain time rather than going for speed.
Sports that have fewer players	Pick one that you like and stick to it.
Add hills or rougher water	Do your homework before embarking on outdoor activities. Heed the ratings systems and come prepared. Never go alone.
More competitive teams	Watch and protect your wrists. Don't go with too heavy a ball.
18 holes and walk the course	Carry your clubs for a better workout.

RESISTANCE TRAINING

To this point in this chapter I've been talking about cardiovascular exercise. The other pillar of health is resistance training.

As I have mentioned, you must include resistance training in your schedule for overall health. These are your years to maintain functionality, so you will want to work your muscles for healthy bones. No need to push hard with heavy weights, but do not go too light, either. Remember, your muscles must be challenged to keep your bones strong and healthy. You may have already begun to lose some muscle mass and bone density, but you can slow the process and in some cases reverse damage with weight-bearing exercise.

What is right for you?

If you lifted weights when you were younger, you probably lifted a variety of weights. If you have been to a gym lately, you may have had to reduce your weights. Don't compare yourself to another time in life; you will only frustrate yourself. You don't have to use traditional weights at all if you don't like. Resistance bands are awesome and come in different tensions. Each color band signifies a different tension. Check with your instructor or trainer to find out which one is right for you.

If you are going to use hand weights, here are some guidelines: a woman may start off with three-pound hand weights. She should be able to increase this to five or six pounds, which is plenty for her goals of functionality. Men are traditionally stronger, because they have more testosterone and more muscle fibers. They should be able to use five- and six-pound hand weights to start and build from there. Men get stronger quicker, but they should also be careful of overdoing it. Remember, you are working toward long-term health.

Partner up

If you are lifting weights outside of the seasoned veterans class, lift with a buddy, even if you are using the machines. In fact, I really don't see the need for you to use free weights at this stage of the game unless it has been a part of your life for a very long time. If you are accus-

174

tomed to free weights, then use them, but I still encourage you to have a partner.

Partners are important for exercises that could harm you, such as the bench press. People have been severely hurt by the bar when they have lost control of it. Be safe, or you could find yourself in trouble. The machines offer a very good workout but are safer overall (if you follow the instructions).

If you work out at a club or fitness center, do not compare yourself to anyone else. No one is the same. We are different ages with different fitness levels and different goals. Remember, small steps for you will do the trick! Any resistance training is better than none. If your muscles have not been worked before, they will be weak. This is a fact. But the exciting news is that your body will respond quickly. Before you know it, you will increase your muscle mass and bone density, both of which are important.

Caution

During any exercise, whether cardiovascular or weight lifting, if you experience pain, stop! Your body is telling you something. It is better to listen up front to your body's whisper than experience it screaming at you later. A little prevention will help you stay at it longer. Pain is often an indicator of too much, too soon.

If you feel pain when doing cardio exercise (muscle pain, not breathing complications), simply reduce your impact, lower your arms, or walk in place. With weight lifting, lower the amount of weight until you eventually build yourself up to a heavier weight. If at any time you experience symptoms remotely close to a heart attack, seek medical attention immediately.

This does not mean you should never feel anything uncomfortable. If you are embarking on a new fitness program, you *will* feel it. You will experience some soreness and muscle fatigue. This is part of the process. If you follow the guidelines in this book, however, such discomfort should be minimal. But nonetheless, it is par for the course when starting a new workout routine.

I mentioned earlier that I highly suggest you seek the counsel of a physician before you start your new program. I can't emphasize this enough, especially if you are overweight or have been living a sedentary lifestyle. If you have a family history of heart disease or other restrictive ailments, you definitely need to get a checkup and overall physical before you begin. Better to be safe than sorry!

Resistance training log

As we recorded your cardiovascular exercise with the activity log, I suggest you record your resistance training on the following log. Besides, this chart ensures that you don't forget a muscle. I spend every day training people, and I still use this log for myself.

Chart 8.5—Resistance Training Log

Muscle	Mode	Seat/ Settings	Weight/ Reps #1	Weight/ Reps #2	Weight/ Reps #3	Stretch?
Quads						
Hamstrings						
Glutes						
Calves						
Inner thigh						
Outer thigh						
Forearms, hands						
Biceps						
Triceps						
Shoulders						
Deltoids						
Pecs						
Lats/ rhomboids						
Erector spinae						
Abs						
Obliques						

WEIGHT-LIFTING EXERCISES FOR SPECIFIC MUSCLE GROUPS

The following pages show you a variety of exercises that you can incorporate into your personal workout. These exercises use a combination of floor work, free weights, and exercise machines. Each one works a major muscle.

Here's to working those muscles to good health!

Quads

You need strong legs in order to have quality of life. They help you get out of bed and handle stairs. An exercise that works the muscles required to do these functional items is a leg lift.

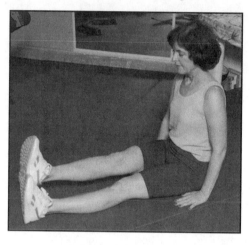

Sit up straight on the floor with your legs out in front of you. (You can also do this sitting in a chair.)

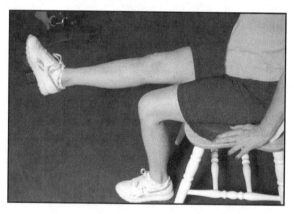

With your hands to your side, lift one leg up, keeping the leg straight but don't lock the knee. You will feel this on the top of your leg or the quad. Slowly lower your leg down and lift the other leg. The key is to go slow and be in control. Breathe out when you lift up.

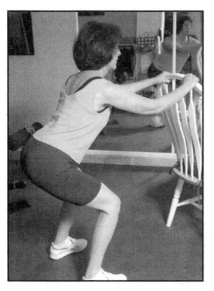

Another great option for your legs is a squat. Get a stable chair (without wheels on it) for this exercise. Your feet should be shoulder-width apart with your feet facing forward. Your legs should not touch the chair, but you are not too far away. Imagine that you are going to sit down in another chair behind you. Push your glute out behind you as if you are trying to sit in the chair. Keep your heels pressed to the floor. As soon as you get close to the "chair" (don't let your bottom touch it), come back up. I like to push my arms out in front of me for counter balance. You can also hold on to another chair, as in this picture. Your knees should never go forward as you do a squat, and you should be able to see your toes.

Hamstrings

We don't want to forget the back of your legs, so here is a good way to curl your legs with an exercise ball. Stand with your left knee pressing into the exercise ball and your right leg at the side of the ball, foot pressing lightly against the ball. In your left hand, hold a pole that touches the floor for a bit of support.

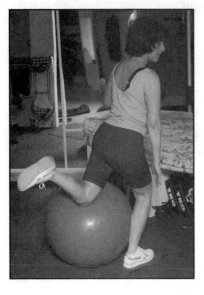

Make sure you are standing as tall as possible, and curl your heel toward your glute, using the hamstring or back of your leg. Curl in, then lower slowly. You may feel a bit unstable—that's actually part of the exercise. You are asking your core muscles, also required for good health, to keep you steady. Breathe out on the curl and in on the lowering of the leg. Switch legs.

You can also do this move without any weight or resistance, as Tim is doing here. Concentrate on making the muscle do what you ask, and you can still get in a good workout.

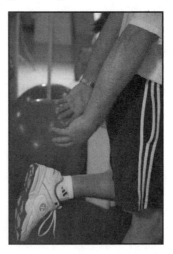

Glutes

To work your glute, I like to use what I call the "table top." You will need to lie down on your back with your knees bent, slightly apart. Your arms will be at your side, and your head comfortable on the floor, looking up at the ceiling.

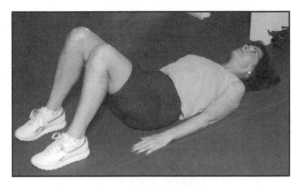

You will lift your glute off the floor, and raise your hip bones toward the ceiling. Lower down, but don't touch the floor. Then repeat. When you lower down, you will be breathing in, and when you are pushing your hips toward the ceiling, you will breathe out.

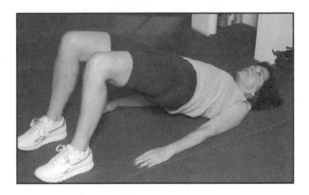

Go nice and slow and work on contracting (squeezing) your glute muscles tight. Feel the burn.

Calves

Your calves are not large muscles such as the quads, hamstrings, and glutes, but they are just as important for walking. Make sure you include calf raises in your routine.

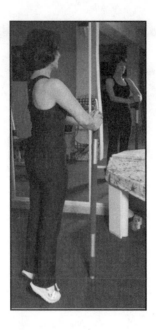

Stand up nice and tall. Have a pole in front of you for support. Do not lean on the pole but simply have it keep you steady. Raise your heels up and stand on your toes. Hold and squeeze this for a few seconds before you lower your heels down. Slow and controlled is the key here.

Also, be sure to lift the toes up (just the opposite movement) to work the front of your calf, as well.

NOTE: After you finish this exercise, take special care as you walk! You may find your feet a bit sluggish to lift for a while, which might make you more inclined to trip.

Inner/outer thigh

Using that same pole, you can work your inner thighs. Once again, stand up nice and tall. Feet are facing forward. Take your right leg out to the side and imagine a ball in front of you. Press the ball toward the middle of your body using your leg. Press and lift back. Breathe out on the press. Switch legs.

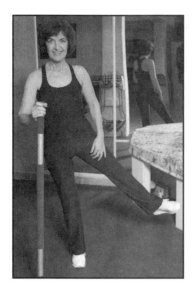 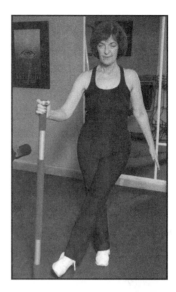

Now to work the outer thigh, sit in a chair. Tie resistance tubing (or exercise band) around your ankles. Feet are facing forward, and you are sitting upright in the chair. Keep your left leg planted on the ground to start, and pull the right leg away. You are using the outside of your leg to pull away. Breathe out on the pull. Switch legs.

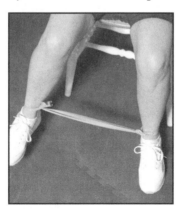

Chapter five has additional ways to work your legs. Keep moving—it's important.

Biceps

Your biceps are important for carrying groceries and holding grandbabies. To work these muscles, grab that resistance band again and take a seat. Place your left hand on your right knee. Then put your right elbow on that left hand. Step on the band (or put your foot through the handle) with your right leg. Grab the other end of the band with your right hand. You start this exercise with the arm down, but don't lock the elbow.

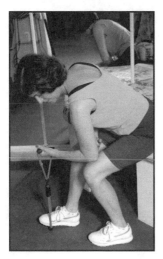

Curl the band up toward you with your right arm. Lower down and curl back up. Breathe out on the curl and in on the lowering phase. You can also do this standing up. Make sure you don't swing and move your back. Make the arm muscle do the work. When you are done with the right arm, switch to the left.

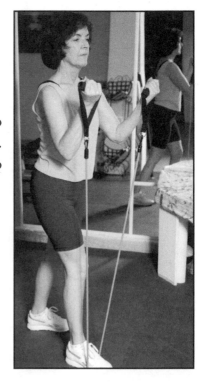

Remember, you can always do traditional curls with hand weights. Be sure to use at least three pounds to get the health benefit.

Triceps

To work the opposing muscle to your bicep, which is the tricep, a great option is what I call "triceps push-ups."

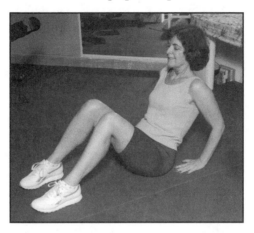

Sit up straight on the floor with your legs out in front of you. Your arms are behind you with your hands/fingers facing toward your body. Be sure to spread your fingers out evenly. Lean back by bending your elbows, and then have the triceps (back of your arm) push you back up. You will also feel this in your abs, but this exercise really concentrates on your arms.

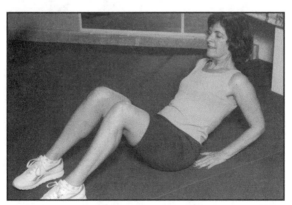

Breathe out as you push yourself up. Don't lock the elbows. You can also work these muscles with an exercise band.

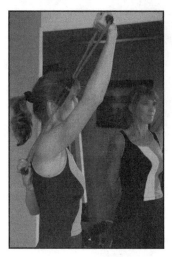

If you have limited shoulder movement, skip this exercise. One arm comes behind to grab the bottom of the band. The opposite arm grabs the band from the top and pulls it up.

Have your hand and wrist facing out, concentrating once again on the triceps. Breathe out as you pull up and in as you lower down. These will help rid you of the flabby or waving arm.

Shoulders and deltoids

For those with limited shoulder movement, you can do a rotator side move. Put a light hand weight in each hand.

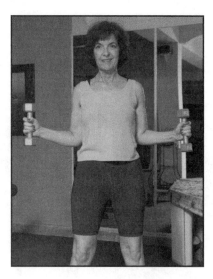

Stand straight, feet forward and knees slightly bent. Place your elbows on your hips. Start with your hands together in front, and move them away from each other.

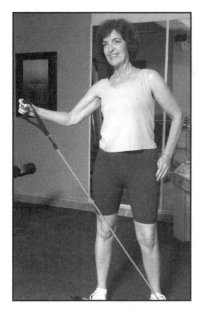

Your arms never lift up. This is a side movement, but it still works the shoulder and deltoids…just without aggravating the rotator cuff. You can do this same move with a resistance band to make it a bit more challenging due to greater range of motion. Step on one end of the band, and pull it away with the opposite arm.

The movement is like pulling a lawn mower string. Start low, and pull up higher. You will raise your arm slightly above the shoulder. If you experience any shoulder pain, lower the range of motion.

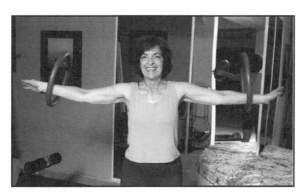

Another great shoulder exercise that can be done with equipment or without is the arm circle. Take your arms out to your side, making a "T" with your arms and body. If you have a set of exercise rings (available at department stores everywhere), then place one on each wrist. The objective is to keep the rings at the wrist line and not let them creep up higher on the arm.

187

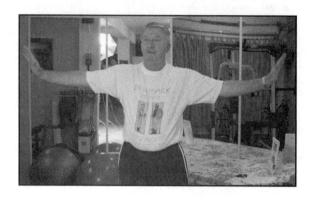

Begin to move your arms forward, making circles. Keep the arms straight, but don't lock the elbows. Continue making circles for twenty seconds. At the conclusion of twenty seconds, change the direction and make small, controlled arm circles backwards. Another twenty seconds here, and you should be feeling it.

Pecs

The older I get, the more I enjoy the variety of exercise equipment out there. The different types of bands have really made some exercises easier on the body yet still very effective. The small band with handles on each side is perfect for a pec pull.

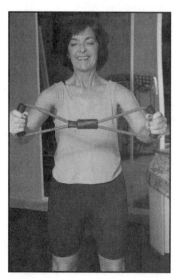

Stand up with your feet forward and knees soft. Bring your arms up in front of you, even with your shoulders. Each hand holds a side of a small band. You will pull your arms away from each other. This really concentrates on the pec muscles. Remember to breathe out on the pull.

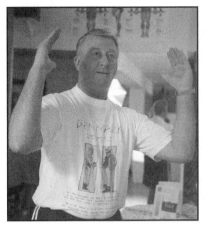

Another option is the traditional butterfly done with or without hand weights. If you do use weights for this exercise, keep the weight light. Your elbows and arms are together in front of you. Keep that 90-degree angle and open your arms up.

Squeeze the arms back together, allowing the elbows to touch. Breathe in as you open up and out as you squeeze.

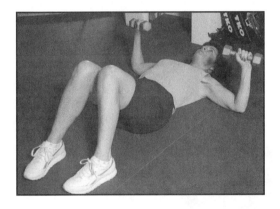

Something else to try is lying on your back on the floor. Make a "U" with your arms, holding hand weights, and then press the weights together to make an "O."

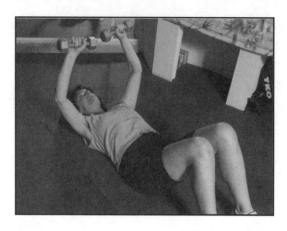

Really squeeze your pec muscles together, and don't lock your elbows. Because you are lying on the floor, you will not be able to lower the arms beyond a good range of motion, so this is a very safe way to work the front of your chest without injuring your back.

Lats and rhomboids

The pecs' opposing muscles are the lats and rhomboids. Using an exercise band, sit on the floor with your legs straight out in front of you. Your legs are flat on the floor, but you don't lock your knees.

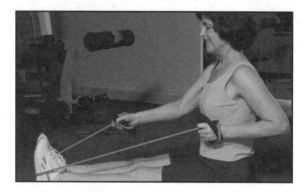

Wrap the band around your feet, with a handle in each hand. Sit up straight as if you have a board on your back. Pull one arm at a time back with your elbow brushing your sides. Pull the other arm. You will alternate each arm.

You can do this same exercise standing up and wrapping the band around a pole.

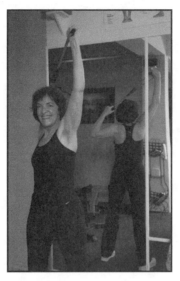

Or you can use hand weights to pull from the floor. Back on all fours with a nice tabletop back. Pull one arm back at a time, elbows brushing your sides. Alternate.

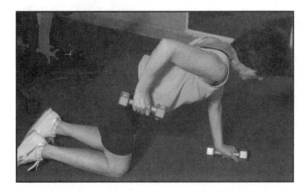

Erector spinae (back)

Although many of the above exercises involve your back, you will still want to isolate and work it. This is one of your core muscles. You need a strong erector spinae.

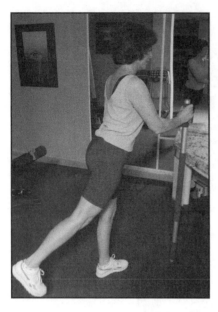

Using a pole or the back of a chair for support, stand up nice and tall. Focus on keeping your upper body straight and aligned while you lift one leg behind you, keeping the leg straight without locking the knee. We are asking the lower back muscle to lift the leg up, so it is *not* important to lift high. Simply make the muscle do what you asked. Watch your posture, and breathe out on the lift.

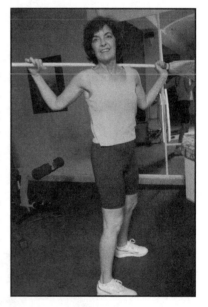

Another option for your lower back is a "torso twist." Using a pole or a broomstick, as Marion is modeling in the photo, place it on the meaty part of your back—by your neck but not *on* your neck. Your arms are behind the pole, and you have a hand on each side. Your legs are slightly bent (soft knees) and your feet are facing forward. The key here is to keep your hips facing forward.

Without moving your hips, rotate your torso to the left, back to center, and then to the right. If you find your hips moving, then you are twisting too hard or too far. You may not have a wide range of motion, but that's OK. The point of this exercise is to work the lower back. In time, you will see improvement. Keep your hips facing forward, and breathe in when you are back to center; breathe out on each side.

Abs and obliques

Another way to prevent back troubles is to work your abs. Since they are opposing muscles, they work together for your back health. Your abs and your erector spinae are your core muscles—arguably the most important muscles in your body.

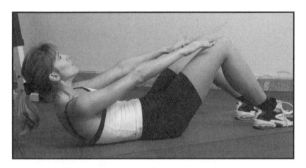

Lie on your back with your knees bent. Anytime you do sit-ups, always have a space between your chin and chest. Picture an apple between your chin and chest, and you'll have the right amount of space. The purpose of this space is to prevent neck strain. You can also focus on aligning your neck with your spine.

Using your abs, sit up as far as you can and tap your knees with your hands. *Hold.* This is not a pulsing movement. This is not a sit-up-and-sit-back-down exercise. This is a contraction. Tap your knees to keep your mind off the fact that your abs are holding you up! Keep tapping. Hold for twenty to thirty seconds, and take a break. Keep breathing in and out throughout your hold. Do not hold your breath.

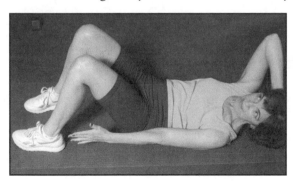

To add a workout for your obliques, lie back down with your knees bent. Place one hand behind your neck. The other arm is straight out by your side. Keeping the arm straight, reach sideways toward your toes. You are aiming for those toes. This is a side-up, not a sit-up. Breathe out as you reach for the toes. Switch sides. Keep your chin away from your chest.

Incorrect posture can hurt your neck and will not work your abs as well. And holding your breath can cause health problems. When you don't breathe, oxygen does not get to your muscles, so they will be weak. When you push your weak, oxygen-deprived muscles, they will demand oxygen that does not exist, and you can get dizzy or even pass out. Obviously this is dangerous, so avoid it simply by breathing.

FUNCTIONAL FITNESS

Whew. I know you have learned how to exercise for your stage of life. Don't let all of the options intimidate you. Start off slow and easy. Incorporate different exercises as you get comfortable, but do something. I encourage you to give them a try. It may take several times before you remember how to properly execute some exercises. Hey, practice makes perfect! Keep looking back at the pictures. It takes time to create new habits, no matter your age.

By concentrating on your workout routine and doing it properly, you are also engaging your mind. Keep this up! Just like our muscles, our minds must be challenged to stay in good shape.

Be safe, and never overdo your exercise or resistance training. Your body will continue to change, but the good news is that you will be ready for it! You are working on functional fitness that will take you the distance.

Here's to not only quantity of life but also quality of life for you!

FIT

Section Four

Nutrition Know-How

50

Chapter Nine

Healthy Food Is Our Friend

Ah, food. What would we do without it? It is the cornerstone of our heritage and the centerpiece of all our traditions. Food is what brings people together. Think back on your favorite memories, and food will most likely be present (weddings, birthday parties, Thanksgiving, Christmas, and so on). I remember as a child eating big, red, ripe tomatoes from our garden like apples, the juice squirting down my clean, white shirt. I was smiling then, and I smile now as I think of it.

Food is comforting. It makes us happy and soothes what ails us. Got a cold? Eat chicken soup. Feeling blue? Have some ice cream. For every mood, a food exists that will make you feel better.

Besides the warm feelings it provides, however, food also has an important purpose: fuel. I am constantly in awe of how God made us. We have the ability to see and record images in our mind forever, viewing them any time we like. We are able to hear an array of intriguing sounds around us and smell the bountiful fragrances. We taste, touch, and feel. We are so complex, yet our "maintenance plan" is so simple: eat right and exercise.

It really is that easy. Good nutrition is the last component of the formula for a long and healthy life. Everything works together: cardiovascular exercise, resistance training, stretching, and proper nutrition. As I stated early on, you have control over 70 percent of the aging process,[1] and this formula is the key.

By honoring the components outlined in this book, you will dramatically influence your metabolism, which, you have probably noticed, may be slowing down a bit. Facts are facts. We cannot lose weight as quickly as we did in our youth.

I love the cartoon I saw many years ago now that showed a woman briskly walking, saying, "Help! Someone is following me!" She turns her head to look behind again and walks even faster. Finally, distraught but disgusted at the same time, she stops. As she turns around, no one is there. In embarrassment, she realizes that what was following her was her big bottom!

Yes, those pounds can follow us. Unfortunately, it is not a laughing matter. The good news is that you can improve your metabolism by eating the right stuff.

FRUIT AND VEGGIE TALES

Your grandchildren may love the veggie characters from the video series VeggieTales, but I am hoping you love the real deal. Fruit and vegetables contain very important vitamins, minerals, and other nutrients that our bodies need to function properly. In fact, in some cases, we cannot get this nutrition anywhere else—certainly not from fast food! God designed us to eat healthy food, not junk food! Think about it: fruit and vegetables are natural foods, not processed. They are 100 percent wholesome. We need to eat these healthy foods if we expect to live a healthy life.

Have you heard the saying, "Garbage in, garbage out"? Computer programmers often use this, but it's also helpful for us to understand what happens with the foods we eat. Our digestive system was not designed for all the chemicals and preservatives that our fast, frozen, and packaged foods contain. If we put unnatural foods in, our digestive track can get clogged. If you are struggling with constipation, chances are that it is your own doing. Try eating more wholesome foods, drinking plenty of water, and exercising.

There is no greater imperative in American health care than switching from a treatment-oriented society to a prevention-oriented society.[2] —Vice Admiral Richard H. Carmona, United States Surgeon General

Many health problems can be treated with better nutrition. In fact, research has suggested that better nutrition is one way that may help prevent 60–70 percent of all cancers.[3] In other words, if people ate better, their bodies would be healthier. If you give your body what it needs, it is much more capable of fighting off disease and illness. But when you deprive it of what it needs, then you are setting yourself up for sickness.

Healthy aging

Jeffrey Blumberg, PhD, associate director at Tufts University's Human Nutrition Research Center, suggests that we eat the following deeply colored fruits and vegetables as often as possible to improve our chances for longevity and health:

- Carrots
- Apples
- Bananas
- Sweet potatoes
- Tomatoes
- Spinach
- Blueberries
- Strawberries
- Broccoli
- Oranges
- Red peppers
- Brussels sprouts[4]

The rule of thumb is the darker the color, the more nutrients the food has in it. Try to eat the entire rainbow, too. God created the rainbow, and He gave foods specific purposes. Each color food contributes a different benefit to the body. It is really quite fascinating when you think about it: natural foods are designed to match our needs.[5]

Drink to your health

Most people aren't drinking enough water throughout the day. This can lead to signs of dehydration, which may include hunger pains and afternoon sleepies. Rather than reaching for a candy bar or taking a nap, try a drink of water instead. Another important reason to drink plenty of water is to maintain the sharpness of our brains, which consist of 80 percent water. Water will help you stay sharp as a tack!

Shades of yellow

Here's a really easy way to evaluate your drinking habits. The next time you urinate, look at the color. If it is a dark color, you are dehydrated and you need to drink water immediately. If your urine is clear, then you are over-hydrated. Believe it or not, you actually don't want to over-hydrate yourself, either. With too much water, you are eliminating most of your nutrients, and you aren't getting the health benefit from them. The perfect color is a very light yellow, which means you are properly hydrated.[6]

I like this tactic better because it is specific to you for *today*. You may have extra salt or sodium one day, and that will impact your hydration. Monitoring the color of your urine is easy to do and helps keep you on track. You will know immediately if you are drinking too much or not enough, and you can correct the problem quickly.

DIETS *Are* TOO GOOD TO BE TRUE

I am sure you have figured it out by now: diets don't work. If they did, we would not need another diet ever again because every single one of us would be "perfectly thin." Don't be misled and think that some pill, drink, powder, or bar will fix your problems.

The so-called diet industry makes billions of dollars each year selling us empty promises. But it takes two to tango, my friend. They sell these things because we buy them! Somehow in our society, we have moved from taking responsibility for our actions to blaming others for our problems. We have forgone "rolling up our sleeves and working hard" in favor of looking for an easy way out. When it comes to obesity (and many other challenges, for that matter), *we* are often the problem.

Though I joked about there being a food to soothe every emotion, eating can be just like any other addiction if we use it to ease our pain or anxiety. Check out the nutritional profile in chapter ten, and ask yourself these questions:

- Does food comfort me?
- Do I eat when I am stressed?
- Do I eat when I am sad, mad, or anxious?
- Do I eat when I am bored?
- Does food enhance/change my mood instantly?
- Do I desperately crave certain foods; do I *have* to have them?

If you relate with any of the above statements, then you may be a stress eater. Stress eating starts with an attempt to cover, mask, or avoid feelings or situations. Although you may feel better temporarily, you're only putting off the inevitable. And besides having the original issue you were contending with, you now feel guilty for overeating, which causes you more pain, then you eat more, and the vicious cycle continues.

If you are a stress eater, I know you desperately want off the spinning wheel. But I caution you: no quick fix exists. You will have to look at your stress, face it, and develop a different approach to it. Exercise can be a great way to replace stress eating.

Buyer beware

NOTE: Many of the weight-loss products you can buy work by causing your body to eliminate enormous amounts of water in a short amount of time. When you lose all that water, the number on the scale *will* go down. Unfortunately, you aren't losing the real problem (fat). All you're losing is water, muscle mass, or both. Water will return, but muscle is harder to rebuild. Plus, if you don't change any of your stress eating or associations with food or behavior patterns, you are most likely going to regain the weight.

You need to understand that the weight-loss industry makes billons of dollars on their quick-fix solutions. They're not really concerned with your health. They just want to make a buck. And because their products don't work, they can sell another one with new promises—which makes them even more bucks. If any of their products really did what they claimed, why would you ever need another weight-loss product?

A client of mine fell for the food replacement bars scam. She thought that if she ate these all day long she would lose weight. Take a look at one of these bars the next time you are in the grocery store. Most of them are extremely high in fat (and calories), especially the ones marked "low carb." They are intended as emergencies, not as meals or snacks.

Here's a tip: When food manufacturers take something out, they will always replace it with greater amounts of something else. Why? We like things that taste good.

Remember this one thing when it comes to food: advertising is all about selling a product. When you see ads for foods, discern what the truth is and don't accept their message as "the whole truth." Buyer beware!

Don't diet

Don't bother dieting, either. Have you ever looked at the rows of diet books at your local bookstore? Egad! If any of them really worked, the rest would be pulled from the shelf. But like weight-loss products, these books are big on claims and low on delivery. Sure, you can find some great nuggets in these diet books, but don't forgo common sense, which is really the only true way to lose weight.

Eating right and exercising represent the only route to good health. Depriving yourself until you feel like you're starving won't help you. Every time you think about what you're not allowing yourself to eat, your mind will be consumed with desire for that thing. I once heard a motivational speaker tell a story about a mother screaming at her kid, who was on the monkey bars, "Don't get hurt! Don't fall." The kid proceeded to fall. He was concentrating on the words "hurt and fall" and, therefore, did just that. The speaker suggested an alternative: "Be careful." The mind then changes focus to "playing with care."

Isn't it funny how our minds work? Tell yourself you can't have something, and that will be all you want. Don't fall for the latest promise to be thin in two weeks. Instead, stick to the tried and true: balance. Balance is God's plan, and as always, His plan is the best. What does His plan look like? I'm glad you asked!

NUTRITION KNOW-HOW

As an advanced personal trainer, I have taken many courses on nutrition. I am happy to provide you with guidance on a well-balanced diet, one that will support a healthy lifestyle for you. If you have a medical condition that requires very specific nutrition, I encourage you to see a certified nutritionist or dietitian about the suggestions in this chapter. These folks have dedicated their lives to proper nutrition and can take what I've outlined to the next level for you. I personally follow these guidelines and have had good success.

I'm sure most of this isn't new to you since the Food and Drug Administration defined a well-balanced diet many, many years ago. Through the years, some minor updates and modifications have been made, and I believe it is still the best route to take. You won't have to give up all your favorite foods or stop living. It will help you make wiser decisions on fueling up your body so that it may run at optimal speed. And if our bodies are operating at their best, we can continue to live life to the fullest.

Here are the basic premise and some guidelines:

Nutrition 101

What you eat must have a mix of carbohydrates, proteins, and fat. The Aerobics and Fitness Association of American, as well most other reputable nutrition institutions, recommends these percentages:

- Carbohydrates = 55–60 percent of diet
- Proteins = 12–15 percent of diet
- Fat = 25–30 percent of diet (no more than 10 percent saturated fat)[7]

Your energy systems that enable you to move and conduct your cardiovascular exercise require carbohydrates. Carbohydrates are the body's main source of energy, and they come in two forms: simple (sugars) or complex (vegetables, grains). They include both sugars and starches.[8]

Low-carb "diets" that dramatically restrict your carb intake are dangerous. Your body *will* get what it needs, one way or the other. If you don't provide what it needs through what you eat, it will take carbohydrates from your organs, most likely your liver. The body will do what it needs to in order to operate. Wouldn't you rather give it what it needs in the proper form and amount?

Fifty-five percent of your diet should be carbohyrdrates.

The good, the bad, and the ugly

Since you may not be as active now and your metabolism is slowing down, I suggest you make carbs 55 percent of your diet. This will be ample for most people. If you are an extreme athlete, then increase it to 60 percent.

The most important factor is ensuring you are eating the *right* carbs. They can be simple or complex, which means they are either easier to digest or a little tougher, respectively. Sugar, candy, cakes, pies, and ice cream are all quickly absorbed into your body, yet they have *zero* nutritional value. This does not make them a good source of fuel. Examples of simple carbs:

- Sugars (natural and processed)
- Fruits
- Some vegetables

Complex carbs move slower into the bloodstream, but they bring with them nutrients required for organ function, movement, thinking, and the like. Examples of complex carbs:

- Potatoes
- Broccoli
- Rice
- Grains
- Carrots
- Corn
- Beans

Refined sugars or processed sugars (found in most junk foods but also in boxed and frozen foods) should be limited to only 10 percent of your total carb intake.[9] Although they will help give you a quick boost of energy, they have no nutritional value. Maybe that's why they call it "junk food." The body will still be craving the nutrition it needs, which is why you feel the need to eat more right away. Your hunger pangs never seem to be satisfied if this is all you're eating.

Super scary

Did you see the movie *Super Size Me?* It is a documentary about a young, healthy man who embarks on an experiment to eat nothing but fast food three times a day for thirty days. At first the greasy food made him sick, but after a while he began to crave it. Before long, he wasn't satisfied with the same amount. His body was "addicted" to junk. Toward the end, his doctors were very concerned that he would have heart failure. He went from a lean, healthy man to a sickly, fat, heart-attack-ready-to-happen. Unbelievable!

Well, not really. When you eat high-fat food such as fast food, the body learns that it doesn't have to burn your stored fat—because it's getting plenty of it in your food. Thus, you gain weight and get fatter. Your body is not working efficiently. You will feel the need to eat more and more (usually a feeling of completely running out of gas) in order to sustain your energy systems. It will not use what it already has stored up, because you trained it not to by providing it junk. And all your excess carbs will be stored as fat.

The Right Carbs

The question really shouldn't be, "Do I eat carbs?" The question should be, "What are the *best* carbs for me to eat?" Focus on that, and you will give your body the energy it needs without packing on the pounds.

Here is a hot list of really nutritionally packed carbs designed to give you energy without the junk:

- Apples
- Oranges
- Peaches
- Pineapples
- Carrots
- Parsley
- Broccoli
- Spinach[10]
- Acerola cherries
- Papayas
- Cranberries
- Beets
- Kale
- Cabbage
- Tomatoes

Try to avoid and/or limit the following when at all possible:

- Soft drinks
- Sugar-filled juices
- Candy
- Cake, cupcakes
- Pies (fruit is a better alternative)
- Ice cream (try soy nondairy frozen desserts instead)
- Muffins, danishes, doughnuts
- Twinkies and other packaged baked items

All Fat Is Not Created Equal

Besides the above foods holding no nutritional value, they are fattening! Let's talk about fat for a minute.

We are very familiar with what too much fat can do to our health. But did you know that our bodies actually *need* fat, just like carbs, for our energy system? Women need a higher percentage of body fat than men for their reproductive system. Fat is what protects you against cold temperatures, acting as an insulator. It is fat that gives your skin and hair a healthy glow. Without enough fat, women can experience amenorrhea or a lack of their menstrual cycle. A lack of fat can also lead to osteoporosis (bone loss), constipation, brittle nails, mood problems, insomnia, and itchy skin.[11]

Twenty-five percent of your diet should be fat.

Like everything else, it is all about balance—eating the *right amount and kinds* of fat. Here are the guidelines:

Twenty-five percent of your total diet should be fat, with no more than 10 percent being saturated fat. Avoid all trans fats, which are even worse than saturated, because they not only increase your bad cholesterol (LDL), but they also lower your good cholesterol (HDL). These fats are a fast-pass to heart disease. Want to lower your risk for heart disease this instant? Give up *all* fried foods! Yes, that includes french fries. Replace fried items with a healthy option such as a salad or steamed vegetables.

Consume the following sparingly:

- Fried foods
- Vegetable oils
- Margarine
- Sweets
- Cheese

Improve good cholesterol

Below is a list of foods that provide the good kind of cholesterol that your body needs or can handle better:

- Olive oil
- Flaxseed oil
- Peanut oil
- Avocados
- Green olives
- Light butter
- Omega-3 fish oils (halibut, salmon, albacore tuna)

As you wean yourself off the wrong types of fatty foods and transition to the better kind, your heart will be much happier!

The next step is to watch your portions.

Watch your portions

Were you raised to clean your plate at dinnertime? Well-meaning parents often create the wrong association with food: eat until it is gone. Instead, we should eat until we are full. We should also take our time when we eat. If we eat fast, our body may not have time to actually tell us it has reached its limits. Slowing down your eating pace can certainly help reduce your portions.

Many people combine the mistake of cleaning their plate with the second mistake of filling it up too high in the first place. Use the palm of your hand as a guide for portion sizes. The smaller your hand, the less you need.

I remember having my grandmother constantly nag me about finishing my plate because there were starving kids in China. Well one day, I'd had enough. I pushed my plate toward her and said, "Here you go, Grandma. FedEx the rest of my dinner to those folks in China. They can have it! I'm full!"

Ever since then I have followed what I call the "skinny person's guide to eating."

The skinny person's guide to eating

Here are some tips that might help your eating habits and move you toward better health.

- Drink a glass of water before you eat.
- Ask for a small or lunch portion (some restaurants even have senior portions, which are smaller, too).
- Share your meal with your friend or spouse.
- Eat your salad first (go easy on the dressing).
- Eat your veggies next.
- Put your fork down as you chew each bite.
- Chew slowly.

- Cut up only one piece of meat at a time.
- Don't eat bread.
- Drink a glass of water midway through your meal.
- Ask for a to-go box before you are finished—this puts pressure on you to actually have leftovers for the box.
- Skip dessert by asking for the check *before* they show you the dessert tray.
- Eat most meals at home where you control the ingredients!

POWERED UP BY PROTEIN

The final thing we need in our diet is protein. We must get enough protein because it's what repairs and restores our muscles. Roughly 12–15 percent of your diet should come from protein. If the intensity of your activities is decreasing, I suggest you lower your protein intake to 12 percent of your diet. If you are exerting yourself, then use the higher end of the range (15 percent).

Twelve percent of your diet should be proteins.

- Protein is vital to your health.
- It builds and repairs body tissues.
- It helps skin, hair, muscles, bones, and teeth.
- It regulates digestion and metabolism.
- It builds antibodies to prevent infection.
- It produces hemoglobin and myoglobin, which transport energy to muscles.
- It makes muscle-contracting proteins called actin and myosin.
- It balances the acidity of the body to aid chemical reactions such as digestion.

- It transports oxygen and other nutrients such as fat and cholesterol.

Many times a protein dish will also include fat. Fat is tricky. It is found in many other foods, so it can sneak up on you. Be careful of the proteins you select. Try these ideas out for meeting your protein needs but keeping the fat content low:

- Beans (also try soy beans)
- Beef (watch the fat content)
- Soy meat substitute
- Cheese (low fat)
- Chicken (skinless)
- Fish (but not fried)
- Milk (choose low-fat or rice/soy with enriched vitamins)
- Tofu

Your target

Now is the time for you to figure out *your* body's requirements for fuel. Use the calorie counter in chapter ten to determine your daily total. The instructions are straightforward, and you will get your CPM (calories per meal) so that you may hit your target meal by meal.

Remember, you are eating to live, not living to eat. Chapter ten also has a great journal that will help you keep track of your daily caloric intake as well as your exercise. It has fantastic resources to help you create a healthy diet and lifestyle. It is there to help—use it!

Chapter Ten

Creating a Healthy Diet

One of the first things my clients ask me for is a target number of calories they should consume every day. Some of them have been using the government's guidelines for daily caloric intake. Please don't! Those guidelines are generic. They suggest that *all* women eat 2,000 calories a day. Well, if I ate that much I'd be fat, and I'm very active!

In this chapter I'll help you design a healthy diet that's right for you. This chapter contains formulas, forms, and other tools for you to create your own healthy diet. Let's start by finding how many calories *you* should be consuming a day.

COUNTING CALORIES

I know that counting calories can take all the fun out of eating for some people, but if we are going to get *in* control of our health rather than *out* of control, it is important to monitor our food intake…at least for a while.

Most food packaging is based upon a 2,000-calorie diet, but most of us don't need to eat that much. You will have to carefully watch labels and begin keeping track of *your* calories. Watch the serving sizes as well. If it has more than one serving, then you have to multiply the calories by the number of servings. Follow the instructions below to find out your CPM (calories per meal). I really like this formula because it takes into account your activity, so you are fueling up exactly right for your lifestyle.

NOTE: To lose weight at a safe rate and ensure the highest possible chance of keeping weight off, women should expect to lose only one to two pounds per week. Men can expect to lose two to three pounds a week.[1] Be realistic and manage your expectations. And remember, muscle weighs more than fat, so as you begin to exercise you may find yourself losing fat but gaining a little weight! That's OK.

Don't get too hung up on a certain weight, but rather know what you want to feel like in certain clothes or aim for a certain clothing size. I personally threw my scale away years ago. I strive for being toned, strong, and fit. I know what size I want to be, and I worry about that more than my actual weight.

FINDING YOUR DAILY CALORIE TOTALS

Having said that, however, I need to also say that calories do matter. We must watch what we take in and aim to burn enough each day.

Use this formula to find how many calories you should be taking in every day. Don't let the math scare you. You can do this.

Current weight (CW) = _____

Record how much you weigh right now. No fudging!

Desired weight (DW) = _____

This is the weight you'd like to get to. I know I just said you should throw your scale out. For this exercise, however, just put down a weight you think you would like to be at. Once you arrive at the size you want, then you can toss the scale!

Difference (DIFF) = _____

In other words, how many pounds do you want to lose? Subtract what you want to weigh (DW) from what you weigh now (CW) and put that number (DIFF) in the blank.

Now we're going to figure out how long it's going to take you to lose that many pounds. The formula is this:

DIFF / PPW = T

DIFF is the number of pounds you want to lose. PPW is the number of *pounds per week* you can safely lose. For women this number is one to two pounds per week. For men it is two to three pounds per week. Let this be your goal for weekly weight loss. Then T (time) is the number of weeks it should take you to drop to your desired weight.

Now you do it:

DIFF _____ pounds divided by PPW _____ pounds per week = T _____ weeks, roughly.

That wasn't too hard, was it? Now you have a feel for how long this will take you. Don't try to rush anything. There aren't any shortcuts to getting fit in a healthy way.

Now let's figure out how many calories you should be taking in. This first formula will determine how many calories you should get per day once you've achieved your desired weight and have settled into a lifestyle of regular exercise. After we find this number, I'll show you how to do one more simple calculation to determine your daily calorie intake to drop those pounds and get to your desired weight.

The formula for *maintaining* your desired weight is this:

DW x 13 = TC

DW, you'll recall, is the weight you want to get to. We'll assume you've settled into a program of *moderate* exercise. That gives us 13 as the number you'll multiply your desired weight by to arrive at your recommended daily caloric intake. (If you were doing more strenuous exercise you could use a higher number, such as 15, and vice versa if you were doing lighter exercise only.) The result of this multiplication is TC, which is the total number of calories you should be taking in per day to maintain your goal weight.

Now you do it:

DW _____ pounds x 13 calories = TC _____ total calories[2]

If you do not wish to lose weight, you're done! This is your daily caloric need. If, however, you still need to get to that desired weight (DW), you must *reduce* your caloric intake per day. All you have to do is take your total from above (TC) and subtract 400 calories, which is a safe yet effective amount to eliminate out of your diet (it's roughly a bagel with cream cheese or a Starbucks grande latte).

TC – 400 = AC

That's your total calories (TC) minus 400 calories a day. The result is your *adjusted calories* (AC). That's how many calories you should be taking in every day to lose your pounds per week (PPW) and get to your desired weight (DW).

Here you go—you're almost there:

TC _____ - 400 calories = _____ adjusted calories (AC)

This is your target per day. Consume this many calories per day, and you will lose weight in a healthy way and on a safe schedule.

To help you get a better handle on what this actually looks like on a daily basis, let's chop up that AC number even smaller. Break it down per meal by dividing by three.

AC _____ divided by 3 meals a day = _____ calories per meal (CPM)

We don't usually eat three evenly balanced meals a day, so you can slide these figures around. Just make sure the total doesn't exceed your AC. Some people don't do the three-meals-a-day thing, preferring up to six smaller meals throughout the day. If that's what you do, simply divide your AC by the number of meals you typically eat in a day. If you eat six meals a day, the formula to find the caloric totals for each meal would be AC divided by 6. Make sense?

The labels on your food packaging will give you calories per serving. Keep a close eye on how big they say their serving sizes are, though. Sometimes they can be tricky.

In the previous chapter, I talked about carbs, protein, and fat. I said your diet should consist of certain percentages of these three main food categories. Here they are again:

- Carbohydrates = 55–60 percent of diet
- Proteins = 12–15 percent of diet
- Fat = 25–30 percent of diet (no more than 10 percent saturated fat)

By using these numbers we can discover how many calories we should get each day from carbs, proteins, and fat. First, we'll do carbs.

If carbs should be 55 percent of your total daily consumption of calories, then we need to find out what 55 percent of your adjusted calories (AC) is.

AC _____ x .55 = _____ carb intake (C)

The recommended range for carbs is 55–60 percent of your diet. We just did the formula for 55 percent. If you want to see what 60 percent would be, simply substitute .60 for .55 in that formula.

I also recommend that you have no more than 10 percent of your carb calories come from what are called processed carbs. That's 10 percent of C, which is already 55–60 percent of AC. In other words, processed carbs should not be more than 5.5–6 percent of your total calories in any given day. To find out what this would be, multiply your C by .1, which is 10 percent.

C _____ x .1 = _____ processed carbs (PC)

Getting lost in the math yet? Hang on—we're almost through!

Twelve to 15 percent of your daily calories should come from proteins. In other words, 12–15 percent of what you eat should be protein.

AC _____ x .12 = _____ protein intake (P)

That's for 12 percent. If you wanted to see what 15 percent would be, substitute .15 for .12 in that formula.

Now let's do fat. You might be surprised that I'm recommending 25–30 percent of your daily diet to be fats. Believe it or not, that's healthy.

AC _____ x .25 = _____ fat intake (F)

For 30 percent, multiply your AC by .3 instead.

Saturated fat should be kept to 10 percent or less of your total fat. This formula will look almost exactly like one for processed carbs. Saturated fat should be 10 percent of your total fat (F), which is already limited to 25–30 percent of your total calories (AC). In other words, calories from saturated fat should not constitute more than 2.5–3 percent of total caloric intake.

F x .1 = _____ maximum saturated fat intake (SF)

There, we're done! Whew. Math isn't my favorite subject either, but now that this is done you have it forever.

Conversion from grams to calories

Thanks to all that math, we've arrived at the daily calorie totals you should get from carbohydrates, protein, and fat. However, your food packaging will not show you these figures in calories, but in grams. Most food packaging will show a calorie total, but when they start breaking it down into fat and cholesterol and the rest, they'll go into grams and milligrams. You need a way to convert the gram totals on the packaging to the calorie totals we've gotten with our math.

It's going to take a little more math, but it's pretty easy. There's one formula for carbohydrates and another for protein and fat.

Every gram of carbohydrates consists of 9 calories.[3] To find out how many *grams* you should get from carbs each day, divide your daily carb calorie total (C) by 9.

C _____ divided by 9 = _____ total number of *grams* from carbs each day (CG)

You can also go the other way. Say you know how many grams of carbohydrates there are in something and you want to know how many calories that will be. Just reverse the formula. Instead of dividing calories by 9, multiply grams by 9. Below, CG is the number of *grams of carbs* an item has, according to the label.

CG _____ x 9 = _____ total number of carbohydrate calories this item has

For example, if your previous math showed that your adjusted calories (AC) for a day should be 1,800, and 55 percent of that should be carbs, you're left with 990 calories that you should get from carbs every day. You turn to your food packaging and find that one serving of a certain item will give you 8 grams of total carbohydrates. So you've got 990 calories on one hand and 8 grams on the other. What do you do?

In this case, you would multiply grams by 9 to find out how many calories of carbs this item will give you: 8 x 9 = 72. One serving of this item will give you 72 calories of carbs, leaving you with a total of 918 calories (990-72) to get from other sources.

Now let's look at how to convert grams to calories when it comes to protein and fat. The key number here is 4, not 9. Every gram of protein or fat has 4 calories.[4] If one serving of an item gives you 13 grams of total fat and 2.5 grams of saturated fat, using the same AC of 1,800, you will receive 52 calories of total fat and 10 calories of saturated fat. If one serving of an item renders 4 grams of protein, it would therefore give you 16 calories of protein. Don't let all the numbers intimidate you. It becomes easier with practice.

NUTRITION AND WEIGHT PROFILE

Below is a quick nutritional profile that will help you evaluate your current eating habits. Please be honest. No one has to see this but you.

Chart 10.1—Nutrition and Weight Profile

Name: _____ Date: _____

What is your current weight? _____

What is your desired weight? _____

If you are trying to lose weight:

What is the MOST you have weighed as an adult? _____

What is the LEAST you have weighed as an adult? _____

What is the lowest weight you have maintained for a year? _____

How many times have you lost and regained weight? _____

What types of "diets" have you tried? _____

If you have high blood pressure or high cholesterol, at what weight did these problems develop? _____

Is this a good time in your life to commit to a weight-loss program? _____

What obstacles are in the way of achieving your goal? _____

Which do you eat regularly (check all that apply):

Breakfast _____   Mid-morning snack _____

Lunch _____   Mid-afternoon snack _____

Dinner _____   After-dinner snack _____

Late night snack _____

How many times a week do you eat out? _____

How many of those times are at fast-food places? _____

What size portions do you normally eat?

Small _____   Moderate _____   Large _____   Supersize _____

How often do you eat more than one serving?

Always _____   Usually _____   Sometimes_____   Never _____

How long does it take you to eat a meal? _____ minutes

Do you eat while doing other activities (e.g. watching TV, reading, working)? Yes/No

How many times each *week* do you eat or drink the following?

_____ Cookies, cake, pie_   _____ Candy

_____ Doughnuts   _____ Ice cream

_____ Muffins   _____ Regular soft drinks

_____ Potato chips, corn chips, etc.   _____ Fried foods

_____ Peanut butter, nuts or seeds   _____ Crackers

_____ Fast food (McDonalds, Taco Bell, Arby's, etc.)

_____ Cheese (including low-fat cheese, cottage cheese)

_____ Whole milk, cream, nondairy creamer

_____ Red meat (beef, pork, lamb)

_____ Butter, margarine, mayonnaise

_____ Breakfast meat or luncheon meat (bacon, sausage, hot dogs, etc.)

_____ Convenience items (frozen foods, instant potatoes, canned items)

_____ Refined grains (white rice, white breads)

_____ More than one serving of alcohol per day (4 oz wine or 12 oz beer)

_____ More than two servings of a caffeinated beverage in a day

How many servings of the following foods do you eat each *day*?

_____ Fruits (fresh)   _____ Vegetables (fresh)

_____ Bread (wheat)   _____ Cereal (whole grain)

_____ Meat

_____ Dairy products (milk, cheese)

_____ Pasta, rice, other grain

_____ Dried beans, peas, tofu, etc.

Use this as a place to start making adjustments. I don't suggest that you try to tackle every bad habit you have all at once. Instead, select one area that you can make improvements on and start today. Can you eliminate fried foods? How about reducing the amount of bread? Remember, by making wiser choices today you can have a healthier tomorrow.

GOOD, BETTER, AND BEST FOOD CHOICES

I know life does not always allow us to make the best choices possible, but we can certainly make *better* choices when it comes to what we eat. Here are some ideas for you to consider when faced with food options.

Chart 10.2—Godd, Better, and Best Breakfasts

GOOD	BETTER	BEST	AVOID
1 bowl canned fruit	1 bowl frozen fruit	1 bowl fresh fruit	Processed sugars
1 Slim Fast breakfast drink	1 Jamba Juice smoothie	Fresh fruit blended with ice and water	High-fat milk products
Fried eggs or omelets	Scrambled eggs	Egg Beaters	Egg yolks (these have twice the cholesterol as meat)
1 English muffin w/ light jam or 1 bagel w/light butter	1 bowl low-sugar, whole-grain cold cereal	1 bowl hot oatmeal with minimal butter and rice milk	Sugary cereals or instant breakfast meals
1 glass fruit juice	V8 low sodium vegetable drink	1 glass freshly squeezed fruit juice or vegetable juice	High-sodium and high-sugar drink
1 Nutri-Grain breakfast bar	1 bran muffin	1 banana and 1 small low-fat yogurt	Foods with high sugar and fat content
1 slice white bread with peanut butter	1 slice whole-wheat bread with light butter	1 slice whole-grain bread with avocado spread	High-fat peanut butter, butter, or sugary jams

NOTE: You can have black coffee, hot tea, or iced tea with breakfast basically calorie-free. You should have on glass of water first thing in the morning to hydrate. And eating one hard-boiled egg (not the yolk) first thing in the morning can set that metabolism for you.

Chart 10.3—Good, Better, and Best Mid-Morning Snacks

GOOD	BETTER	BEST	AVOID
1 Nutri-Grain breakfast bar	Handful of dried fruit and nuts	1 apple, banana, orange, tangerine, or plum, etc.	Sweet rolls, doughnuts, muffins
1 glass fruit juice	Protein drink (soy based or veggie based)	Hard-boiled eggs (whites only)	Yolks, whey products, and sugary drinks

NOTE: If you had protein for breakfast, you probably will not need it mid-morning. Remember, we often take in too much protein. Watch yourself carefully here. But if you had only gruit and grains, you might consider a protein option here. Have some water.

Chart 10.4—Good, Better, and Best Lunches

GOOD	BETTER	BEST	AVOID
Jack in the Box or other fast-food oriental chicken salad (go light on dressing)	Grocery store packaged salad mix	Freshly made green salad with crab, or fresh salad bar	Fried chicken slices, heavy/creamy dressings; skip the bread or crackers.
Egg salad sandwich with light mayo	Tuna sandwich with light mayo	Turkey sandwich with no mayo	Wheat bread or low-fat white alternative. Check labels. Replace chips with veggies or pretzels.
Jack in the Box teriyaki chicken bowl or other rice bowl	Canned vegetable, turkey, or bean soup, low sodium	Homemade bowl of vegetable, turkey, or bean soup	Anything with heavy sodium. Limit crackers and bread.
Ham and cheese sandwich	Grilled chicken breast sandwich	Veggie burger	Heavy sauces, any fried sides, and too much bread; again, try fruit or veggies on the side instead.
2 tacos	Baked potato with light butter and fresh mushrooms only	Fresh veggie wrap	Large amounts of butter, sour cream, and cheese
Carl's JR "Low Carb" burger; no fries	McDonald's Veggie Burger; no fries	Homemade soy burger; no fries	Avoid the buns, heavy sauces, and cheese.

NOTE: Go light on the bread if you had bread in the morning. If you did not have any grains in the morning, then bread is fine at lunch. Remember, bread is considered a processed sugar unless it consists mostly of grains. Beware: Not all wheat breads are created equal. Some of them are even higher in sugar than white bread. Watch the labels. Whenever possible, replace fried or questionable sides with fruit or vegetables. Have some more water.

Chart 10.5—Good, Better, and Best Afternoon Snacks

GOOD	BETTER	BEST	AVOID
Fruit Roll-Up or fruit bar	1 apple, banana, orange, tangerine, or plum, etc.	Carrots or celery sticks	Processed sugars
1 handful of baked chips, light salt	1 handful of pretzels	Lightly salted or no-salt almonds, walnuts, or pecans	Anything with high sodium
3 pieces candy or chocolate	Handful of trail mix or dried fruit	Sugar-free gum or dry whole-grain cereal	Anything with high-fat content

NOTE: If you had sugar in your breakfast or lunch (juice included), go easy on the sugar now. Natural sugars such as fruit can usually satisfy the craving. Drink more water.

Chart 10.6—Good, Better, and Best Dinners

GOOD	BETTER	BEST	AVOID
Boxed/frozen fish (not fried) with canned veggies	Frozen fish packages in seafood section with frozen veggies	Fresh fish with fresh veggies	Fried fish and heavy sauces; watch condiments
1 chicken fajita with baked chips	1 soy burger on wheat bun with broiled potato slices	1 skinless, boneless broiled chicken breast with brown rice	Skin-on chicken
Grilled pork chop with mashed potatoes	1 broiled turkey leg with low-sugar apple sauce	1 piece soy meatloaf with steamed vegetables	Fatty meat
1 small bowl spaghetti or other pasta in light sauce	1 piece lean steak with baked yam	Baked potato with grilled chicken slices	Bread, fatty cuts of meat; watch condiments
Wendy's chili and side salad	Canned soup and packaged salad, light dressing	Homemade soup, homemade salad with vinegar dressing	Bread
2 slices cheese pizza with a side salad, light dressing	Angel hair pasta with vegetables, side salad, light dressing	Chef salad, light dressing	Alcohol, bread

NOTE: I did not list it because it is a big jump for most, but steamed squash (acorn, butter, or spaghetti) make very nutritious meals combined with a nice salad. Have a small dinner salad with any option with light dressing. Again, if you have already had bread earlier in the day, try to avoid it at dinner.

Chart 10.7—Good, Better, and Best Evening Snacks

GOOD	BETTER	BEST	AVOID
1 frozen fruit bar	Soy ice cream	Fresh fruit	High-fat items
1 handful of pretzels	1 handful of trail mix or dried fruit	1 cup almonds, walnuts, or pecans; no salt	High-sodium items
3 pieces candy or chocolate	Popcorn with light butter and light or no salt	Rice cakes	Big portions
1 glass fruit or vegetable juice	Carrots or celery sticks	1 apple, banana, orange, tangerine, or plum, etc.	Sugary items
Slice of cake	Slice of "sugar-free" cake	Slice of angel food cake with strawberries (no whip cream)	High-calorie, low-nutrition foods

It is OK to be "bad" for up to four meals a week if you use the 80/20 rule (see below), but try to be good the other days. If you cannot be trusted with sweets around the house, then don't buy them!

Carbs have gotten so much attention in the last year or so. Besides eating the right ones, people often wonder *when* they should eat them. A quick reference for you is this: since carbs are fuel or energy for your body, eat them prior to exercise, like the night before. And since muscles require *protein* to recover, eat your protein after working out.

You may have been told to taper your carbs as the day goes. If you have arthritis or similar conditions, this might work for you. Eat your protein at night so that your muscles can repair while you sleep (our muscles are 80 percent water and 20 percent protein).[5] If you are very active, you may do just fine with eating some carbs at night. Test it out, and find out what makes you feel the best.

The food items I've suggested above are not intended to be eaten all at once. These are just ideas for you to consider. I'm sure you'll come up with other options. The more you have, the better your choices, and that will get you healthier.

Quick tips

Quick ways to make better food choices TODAY:

- Opt for healthy side dishes instead of fried ones.
- Choose fresh over frozen, and frozen over canned or boxed.
- Pick bright, rich-colored vegetables, and don't over-cook them. (The more color the vegetable has, the more nutrients for you.)
- Select lean cuts of meat.
- Avoid hot dogs, unless they are 100 percent lean turkey meat.
- Reduce portion sizes.
- Limit bread, and select whole-grains over white or traditional wheat.
- Avoid processed and pack-aged foods, and replace with natural, whole foods.
- Limit your dairy intake; switch to no-fat milk or rice milk.
- Make homemade meals when possible.
- Read food packaging labels carefully.

Travel tips

When you travel, you may find it more difficult to eat right. Here are some suggestions for eating right when you're on the road:

- Eat breakfast bars rather than big, greasy breakfasts out.
- Pack dried fruit as it does not go bad.
- Bring plenty of water bot-tles.
- Pack trail mix.
- Bring Fruit Roll-Ups.
- Have a bag of pretzels handy.
- Stay in places that have a kitchen, and cook your own meals.
- Share meals, and get an extra salad.
- Eat lots of salads.
- Say no to dessert, or opt for sherbet or fresh fruit.
- Don't eat too late (usually not past 7:00 p.m., if possi-ble).
- Keep portion sizes small.
- Don't clean your plate.

Food calorie calculator

Here's a quick guide to how many calories there are in some common foods.[6]

Chart 10.8—Food Calorie Calculator

FOOD	TOTAL CALORIES
Bagel without cream cheese	77
Bagel with cream cheese	340
Nutri-Grain breakfast bar	143
Cranberry juice	137
McDonald's Chicken Caesar Salad w/o dressing	210
Jack in the Box Chicken Caesar Salad with dressing	628
Subway 6-inch tuna sandwich on wheat bread	350
Fresh salmon	174
Meatloaf, 3 oz.	205
1 piece licorice	30
Movie theater popcorn, medium, w/butter	1,170
Movie theater popcorn, medium, w/o butter	900
Popcorn at home made with oil, 1 cup	55
Microwave popcorn, light, 1 cup	25

For more calorie estimates of the foods you are eating, go on the Internet to www.calorieking.com. This Web site allows you to find the calories for many brand-name foods and menu items in restaurants, and it adjusts to the portion size. In addition, it provides information on nutrition (fat, carbs, and percentages of total calories). Just remember that these percentages will be based upon a 2,000-calorie diet. Refer back to your individual total you calculated and adjust accordingly.

FOOD BANK

Do you remember learning the food pyramid in school? Although it has been around forever, it still works. I have another system I call the food bank. It is a great way to show you how you can get the right amount of nutrition in per week.

I like to train people to think of their calories as money in a bank account. You start off each day with a full account by category. As you eat, you deduct amounts out of your food bank just as you would a checking account. When you run out of funds in your checking account, you're broke, right? The logical thing to do then is to stop spending money. Apply this same basic principle to your eating habits. When you're out of "points," stop eating!

Most diets work in just the opposite manner. You are adding your way up to your total. I believe we are more accustomed to subtracting, so I think this will work better for you.

Here is a food bank with descriptions to give you an idea of how you can "spend" your points (notice that this forms a food pyramid of sorts, too):

Chart 10.9—Food Bank Servings

CATEGORY	SERVINGS	DESCRIPTION
Sweets	5 per week	1 cup low-fat yogurt, $^1/_2$ cup frozen yogurt, 1 Tbsp. sugar, syrup, or jam
Beans, nuts, seeds	7 per week	$^1/_2$ cup beans, $^1/_3$ cup nuts, 2 Tbsp. sunflower seeds
Oils/dressing/mayo	14 per week	1 Tbsp. oil, 1 tsp. mayo or 2 tbsp. low-fat mayo, 1 Tbsp. salad dressing or 2 Tbsp. light salad dressing
Low-fat dairy	14 per week	1 cup low-fat milk or yogurt, $1^1/_2$ oz. cheese
Seafood/poultry/ meat	14 per week	3 oz. broiled or roasted seafood, skinless poultry, or lean meat
Whole grains	56 per week	1 slice bread, $^1/_2$ cup dry cereal, $^1/_2$ cup cooked rice or pasta or cereal
Veggies and fruit	70 per week	1 cup lettuce or $^1/_2$ cup other veggies, 1 medium fresh fruit or $^1/_2$ cup frozen or canned fruit, $^3/_4$ cup fruit juice[7]

Calories, like costs, can add up quickly. As with our real bank accounts, our food bank points go fast. Keep an eye on your deductions. The good news is that fruit and veggies are so low in calories that it is like spending pennies. It takes way more of these to add up than the high-ticket items such as junk food and fast food.

Below is a sample bank account for you. You can print it out or scan it and add it to your computer or PDA. However it works for you, keeping track of your "spending" will ensure you don't overdraw. If you have ever used Weight Watchers, they believe in counting points as well. They count up, but the concept is similar. Either way, you must stay within your points for the day.

Chart 10.10—Food Bank Record

Category	Svgs	Mon	Tues	Wed	Thurs	Fri	Sat	Sun	Total
Sweets	5								
Beans, nuts, seeds	7								
Oils, dressing, mayo	14								
Low-fat dairy	14								
Seafood/poultry /meat	14								
Whole grains	56								
Veggies, fruits	70								
TOTAL									

THE 80/20 RULE

Another way of keeping track of what you eat in a week is a principle I call the 80/20 rule. This is what I live by. If you came from the corporate world or were involved in sales, you are quite familiar with the idea that 80 percent of your business comes from 20 percent of your customers. I like to apply this to my eating habits.

Here's how the 80/20 rule works: eat the healthiest you can 80 percent of the time, and don't worry about the rest.

You're going to have "oops" meals and emergency meals. That's part of life. The 80/20 rule is a realistic and flexible plan for eating well.

If you eat three meals a day seven days a week, you will eat 21 meals a week. To apply the 80/20 rule we have to know what 20 percent of that is. Thus: 21 (meals) x .2 (20 percent) = 4.2 (meals). For simplicity, we'll round this down to 4.

So if you eat seventeen healthy meals a week, you have four meals to "blow." If you have a party or special occasion, use one of these four meals to cover them. This way, you are allowing life to happen.

The guidelines for the 80/20 rule are as follows. For your seventeen meals (80 percent of the time):

- Avoid all fried foods.
- Avoid all white and wheat bread (regular wheat is just as bad; whole grains are OK).
- Avoid all sweets (candy, cookies, cake, ice cream, jam, juices).
- Avoid all junk food (boxed, bagged, etc.; try no-salt nuts instead).
- Avoid fast food.
- Avoid alcohol.
- Avoid fatty foods (watch meat portions).
- Avoid whole milk products (use rice or soy).
- Limit cheese intake.
- Watch salt.
- Eat tons of veggies.
- Eat a lot of fruit.
- Drink your water.

For your four meals (20 percent of the time) you may choose to:

- Eat bread (in moderation).
- Eat sweets (in moderation).
- Eat junk food (in moderation).
- Still limit cheese.
- Consume alcohol (in moderation).
- Eat fast food (make wise choices).

I encourage you to give the 80/20 rule a try. Unlike the restrictive trendy diets, it is realistic and allows you to live a little. Be careful, though, and don't load up all your "bad meals" at once. You will never get ahead this way. The bottom line is to make one good choice after another. Each no you say to junk food is a step closer to better health. And with each no, you will gain strength and confidence. Before you know it, you will be eating right and living well as a matter of habit!

DAILY HEALTH JOURNAL

I know that recording your eating habits is probably the last thing you want to do, but it may be the very thing you need in order to get a grip. I encourage you to reproduce the following journal page and use it every day for at least thirty days.

You will be amazed at how it will affect your decisions when you have to actually write down what you're eating and drinking. Even better is to share your journal with someone who will review it and hold you accountable. That is where a personal trainer can really benefit you. A personal trainer would become your accountability partner to encourage you on your journey to better health. Since I can't personally meet with you, this journal can serve as an extension of me. It looks at your entire life, helping to keep you on track.

Chart 10.11—Daily Health Journal

Date:_____

BREAKFAST = _____Calories per Meal (CPM)

Quantity   Food   Calories   Time of Day

SNACK = _____CPM Hungry? ☐ Bored? ☐ Stressed? ☐

Quantity   Food   Calories   Time of Day

LUNCH = _____CPM Alone? ☐ Friend/Family? ☐ Work? ☐

Quantity   Food   Calories   Time of Day

SNACK = _____CPM Hungry? ☐ Bored? ☐ Stressed? ☐

Quantity   Food   Calories   Time of Day

DINNER = _____CPM Out? ☐ Home? ☐ Stressed? ☐

Quantity   Food   Calories   Time of Day

TOTAL CALORIES FOR THE DAY =

I was: Right on Track ☐   Over Daily Total ☐   Under ☐

What adjustments can be made for tomorrow? _____

"Beautiful young people are accidents of nature.
But beautiful old people are works of art."

Cardio Exercise Today:

Activity: _____

Length of Time: _____

Estimated Calories Burned: _____

Did I stretch? Yes ☐   No ☐

How do I feel? Great! ☐   Good ☐   Fair ☐   Poor ☐

Resistance Training Today:

Upper Body ☐   Lower Body ☐   Both ☐

Length of Time: _____

Estimated Calories Burned: _____

Did I stretch? Yes ☐   No ☐

Spiritual Health:

Activity: _____

Length of Time: _____

Mental Health: Did I read today? Yes ☐   No ☐

Prescriptions & Supplements Taken: _____

Water Intake:
(8 oz. Glasses) ☐   ☐   ☐   ☐   ☐   ☐   ☐   ☐

# of Hours of Sleep I Got Last Night: _____

Meal Planning

One way I take control of my nutrition is by planning out my week and buying the appropriate groceries for the week. I shop only once, and I buy only what I need. Select a day that you can review your calendar and upcoming events. Then map out the necessary meals for the week ahead. Write down the ingredients you will need and buy only those items. Be careful of "buy 10, get 1 free" specials. Usually you don't save that much, and now you have way more food than you need. Extra food only becomes a temptation.

A great Web site that provides awesome recipes is www.mealsmatter .org. You will need to register, but they don't ask for any inappropriate information. You can opt out of newsletters and simply utilize the recipe database. They have a *healthy* button with recipes that are healthier. Take a look, be creative, and have fun!

May Good Health Be Yours

Each step you take toward health is a victory. Focus on what you have done right and what changes you can make the next day to be even better. The Healthy Life Journal is really a great tool for taking each day as it comes but looking ahead to tomorrow. Don't lose sight of why you are doing this. Remember, God loves you as you are today, but the healthier you are the more you will be able to do for Him. Keep pressing on!

Conclusion

The Life You Deserve

I hope our journey together through this book has been informative and encouraging for you. We have learned a lot together about the next stages of life, discovered some new truths, and now have a foundation upon which to build your new, healthy lifestyle. My prayer is that you do make changes that will improve your health and increase the quality of your life.

Good health isn't something that happens in one day. You can't buy it on television or order it from a catalog. It is a lifelong commitment.

One of my fitness students commented the other day on how I stay the same, year after year. I don't gain and lose weight; I remain the same. He asked how I do it. My reply was simply that I apply what I teach. I eat right and exercise every day. It is not a fad or trend for me. I choose to live a healthy life today so that I have more tomorrows that will be bright and happy. I want the same for you.

I want to leave you with a poem I wrote some years ago, but I pray it encourages you today. Thank you so much for allowing me to be a part of your life. I truly wish you a very bright and healthy tomorrow!

THE LIFE YOU DESERVE

Life is crazy with its twists and turns.
It can sting you like a bee and really burn.

Life brings to us challenges and obstacles to overcome.
It is stressful and overwhelming to some.

Stress can turn to illness in an attempt to defeat.
That is why your stress you must beat.

If you don't take charge of your life, no one else will.
You must be prepared for the climbs uphill.

Luck is preparation meeting opportunity in your life.
The more prepared you are, the less strife.

Do whatever it takes to manage well.
Your final outcome, only time will tell.

But you will become a healthier you.
You will be less stressful no matter what you do.

You deserve a happier life, don't you know?
Let love, joy, and peace be what you show.

Balanced living is what it is all about.
You were intended for much more, have no doubt.

Don't settle for less and accept that stress.
Don't assume that your life will always be a mess.

Do whatever you need to do.
You're the only you!

May God bless you as you make different choices.
May you always hear only uplifting and encouraging
    voices.

May you be strong when times are tough.
May you know that what you have is already enough.

May good health be your goal.
May you have it right with God and your soul.[1]

NOTES

INTRODUCTION
LIFE'S BEST CHAPTER

1. Johnnie Godwin, *How to Retire Without Retreating* (Uhrichsville, OH: Barbour Publishing, 2005).
2. Aerobics and Fitness Association of America, Advanced Personal Trainer Certification, September 20–21, 2003, San Diego, CA.
3. Ibid.
4. JoAnn E. Manson, MD, PhD, et. al., "The Escalating Pandemics of Obesity and Sedentary Lifestyle: A Call to Action for Clinicians," *Archives of Internal Medicine* 164 (February 2004): 249–258.
5. Mary Yoke, MA, *A Guide to Personal Fitness Training,* ed. Laura A. Gladwin, MS (Sherman Oaks, CA: Aerobics and Fitness Association of America, 2001), 6.
6. David Schwartz, *Speaker's Sourcebook II,* (Englewood Cliffs, NJ: Prentice Hall, 1994), 345.
7. Aerobics and Fitness Association of America, Advanced Personal Training Conference, September 20–21, 2003, San Diego, CA.
8. Aerobics and Fitness Association of America, Cycling Certification, February 12, 2005, Los Angeles, CA.

CHAPTER 2
YOU MAKE THE DIFFERENCE

1. Anthony Robbins, *Unlimited Power* (New York, NY: Ballatine Books, 1986), 200.
2. Henry Cloud and John Townsend, *Boundaries* (Grand Rapids, MI: Zondervan Publishing, 1992).
3. Lorraine Bossé-Smith, *A Healthier, Happier You: 101 Steps for Lessening Stress* (Uhrichville, OH: Barbour Publishing, 2004).

CHAPTER 3
THE TRUTH ABOUT AGING

1. Alliance for Aging Research, "Adding Luster to Your Golden Years," *Living Longer and Loving It!,* Summer 2002, http://www.agingresearch.org/living_longer/summer_02/feature/feature.htm (accessed February 21, 2005).
2. Ibid.
3. Daniel J. Levinson, *The Seasons of a Man's Life* (New York: Ballantine Books, 1986), 33.
4. Alliance for Aging Research, "Detecting Depression Before It's Too Late," *Living Longer and Loving It!,* Spring 2004, http://www.agingresearch.org/living_longer/spring_04/depression.cfm (accessed February 21, 2005).
5. Heidi Haller, "Ageless Milestones," *Under the Sun,* December 2004, 17.
6. Alliance for Aging Research, "Detecting Depression Before It's Too Late."
7. Alliance for Aging Research, "Adding Luster to Your Golden Years."
8. Nancy S. Cetel, MD, *Double Menopause* (New York: Wiley, 2002).
9. Melinda Fouché, *Brain Fitness* (Murrieta, CA: February 9, 2005).

10. Alliance for Aging Research, "The Costs of Being a Woman!", *Living Longer and Loving It!*, Winter 2003, http://www.agingresearch.org/living_longer/winter_03/costofwomen .cfm (accessed February 21, 2005).

CHAPTER 4
THE TRUTH ABOUT CARDIOVASCULAR EXERCISE

1. Brian J. Sharkey, PhD, *Fitness and Health* (Champaign, IL: Human Kinetics, 1997).
2. Aerobics and Fitness Association of America, Advanced Personal Training Conference, September 20–21, 2003, San Diego, CA.
3. Yoke, *A Guide to Personal Fitness Training*, 29.
4. Aerobics and Fitness Association of America, Advanced Personal Trainer Conference, September 20–21, 2003, San Diego, CA.
5. Peg Jordan, RN, *Fitness Theory and Practice* (Sherman Oaks, CA: Aerobics and Fitness Association of America, 1997), 176.

CHAPTER 5
THE TRUTH ABOUT WEIGHT-BEARING EXERCISE

1. Jordan, *Fitness: Theory and Practice*, 110.
2. Lorraine Bossé-Smith, *Finally FIT!* (Lake Mary, FL: Siloam, 2004).
3. Aerobics and Fitness Association of America, Advanced Personal Trainer Conference, September 20–21, 2003, San Diego, CA.
4. Ibid.
5. Jordan, *Fitness: Theory and Practice*, 126–127.
6. Ibid., 56.
7. Ibid., 126–127.
8. Aerobics and Fitness Association of America, Aerobics Instruction Primary Certification, August 25, 2001, Camarillo, CA.

CHAPTER 7
FOCUSED FITNESS FOR FIFTY-SIX TO SIXTY-FIVE-YEAR-OLDS

1. Author unknown.
2. "The Full Retirement Age Is Increasing," Social Security Online, http://www.ssa.gov/pubs /ageincrease.htm (accessed October 6, 2005).

CHAPTER 8
FUNCTIONAL FITNESS FOR SIXTY-SIX AND OLDER

1. *Taste for Life*, March 2005, 16.

CHAPTER 9
HEALTHY FOOD IS OUR FRIEND

1. Aerobics and Fitness Association of America, Personal Training Certification, September 20–22, 2002, San Diego, CA.
2. "Reshaping America's Health Care for the Future," testimony of Richard H. Carmona, MD, MPH, FACS, Surgeon General, before the Joint Econnomic Committee, United States Congress, October 1, 2003, http://www.hhs.gov/asl/testify/t031001a.html (accessed October 7, 2005).

3. "New Survey of American Uncovers Widespread Fear of Cancer, but Little Knowledge About Reducing Risk," American Institute for Cancer Research (AICR) Press Release, July 17, 2001, http://www.aicr.org/press/pressrelease.lasso?index=1318 (accessed October 7, 2005).

4. Jeffrey Blumberg, PhD, "One Serving of Youth, Please," *Living Long and Loving It!,* Winter 1999, http://www.agingresearch.org/living_longer/winter_99/feature/feature.htm (accessed February 21, 2005).

5. Paulette Suzanne, BA, CNC, "The Rainbow Diet" (workshop, Temecula, CA, October 5, 2004).

6. Aerobics and Fitness Association of America, Cycle Certification, February 12, 2005 Los Angeles, CA.

7. Jordan, *Fitness: Theory and Practice,* 225–228.

8. Yoke, *A Guide to Personal Training,* 93.

9. Jordan, *Fitness: Theory and Practice,* 228.

10. "Family Nutrition Made Simple," *Juice Plus,* September 2004.

11. Jordan, *Fitness: Theory and Practice,* 228.

CHAPTER 10
CREATING A HEALTHY DIET

1. Jordan, *Fitness: Theory and Practice,* 244.

2. Ibid.

3. Carol L. Otis, MD, "Fat Figures: How Many Grams of Fat Make Up 20 Percent of Your Calories," Sports Doctor.com, http://www.sportsdoctor.com/articles/fat_figures.html (accessed August 15, 2005) as quoted in Carol L. Otis, MD, and Roger Goldingay, *The Athletic Woman's Survival Guide* (N.p.: Human Kinetics Publishers, 2000).

4. Ibid.

5. Aerobics and Fitness Association of America, Advanced Personal Training Certification, September 20–21, 2005, San Diego, CA.

6. Food Database, CalorieKing.com, http://www.calorieking.com (accessed March 31, 2005).

7. Jordan, *Fitness: Theory and Practice,* 230–231.

CONCLUSION
THE LIFE YOU DESERVE

1. Lorraine Bossé-Smith, "The Life You Deserve."

BIBLIOGRAPHY

Blumberg, Jeffrey, PhD. *One Serving of Youth, Please.* www.agingreserach.org. Winter 1999.

Bossé-Smith, Lorraine. *A Healthier, Happier You: 101 Steps for Lessening Stress.* Uhrichsville, OH: Barbour Publishing, 2004.

———. *Finally FIT! Customizing Fitness to Your Personality Type.* Lake Mary, FL: Siloam, 2004.

Carmona, Vice Admiral Richard H., MD, MPH, FACS. *Juice Plus Newsletter.* Memphis, TN: NSA, March 31, 2005.

Cetel, Nancy S., MD. *Double Menopause.* New York: Wiley, August 2002.

Cloud, Henry and John Townsend. *Boundaries.* Grand Rapids, MI: Zondervan Publishing, 1992.

Dorfman, Lisa. *The Tropical Diet: a Scientific, Simple, and Sexy Weight Loss Strategy for Health, Sport, and Life.* N.p.: Food Fitness International, June 2004.

Family Nutrition Made Simple. Memphis, TN: Juice Plus/NSA, September 2004.

Fouché, Melinda. *Brain Fitness.* Murrieta, CA: The Fouché Institute, February 9, 2005.

Godwin, Johnnie G. *How to Retire Without Retreating.* Uhrichsville, OH: Barbour Publishing, 2000.

———. *Life's Best Chapter.* Birmingham, AL: New Hope Publishers, 1996.

Jordan, Peg, RN. *Fitness Theory and Practice.* Sherman Oaks, CA: Aerobics and Fitness Association of America, 1997.

Levinson, Daniel J. *The Seasons of a Man's Life.* New York: Ballantine Books, 2001.

Manson, JoAnn E., MD, PhD, Patrick J. Skerrett, MS, Philip Greenland, MD, and Theodore B. VanItallie, MD. "The Escalating Pandemics of Obesity and Sedentary Lifestyle: a Call to Action for Clinicians." *Archives of Internal Medicine,* February 2004.

Schwartz, Dr. David. *Speaker's Sourcebook II.* Englewood Cliffs, NJ: Prentice Hall, 1994.

Sharkey, Brian J., PhD. *Fitness and Health.* Champaign, IL: Human Kinetics, 1997.

Smith, Hyrum W. *The 10 Natural Laws of Successful Time and Life Management.* New York: Warner Books, 1994.

Suzanne, Paulette, BA, CNC. *The Rainbow Diet.* Temecula, CA: Juice Plus, October 05, 2004.

Swindoll, Charles. *Laugh Again.* Nashville, TN: W Publishing, reprint edition, 1995.

Taste of Life. March 2005.

Under the Sun. December 2004.

Van Roden, Julie. *A Guide to Personal Fitness Training.* Sherman Oaks, CA: Aerobics and Fitness Association of America, 1997, 2001.

Worley, Karla. *Growing Weary Doing Good?* Birmingham, AL: New Hope Publishers, 2001.

www.agingresearch.org. "Adding Luster to Your Golden Years." Alliance for Aging Research, 2000, 2002.

———. "Detecting Depression Before It's Too Late." Alliance for Aging Research, 2004.

———. "Living Longer and Loving It!" 2003.

www.factfinder.census.gov. Washington, DC: U.S. Census Bureau, 2000, 2002.

Stay on the path to good health

We pray that you have been motivated and energized with Fit Over 50. Lorraine Bossé-Smith shares an upbeat message with everyone she encounters, and this book is no exception.

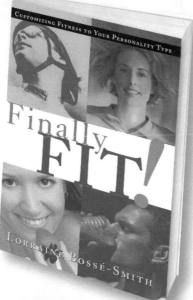

$13.99 / 1-59185-416-4

Imagine a fitness program that is either fast, fun, friendly, or factual—one that fits you. Now you can discover your FIT (Fitness Individuality Trait) using an exclusive personality assessment program.

Your fitness journey features a customized, unique exercise program that will revolutionize your life.

Visit your local bookstore.
Call 800-599-5750
Go to www.siloam.com and save 25%
Mention Offer: BP6101

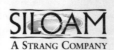